WEIGHT LOSS, ITALIAN STYLE!

Ditch the Diet, Pass the Pasta, and Drop the Pounds FOREVER

Jill Hendrickson

New York

Weight Loss, Italian-Style!
Ditch the Diet, Pass the Pasta, and Drop the Pounds FOREVER

Cover photo by Michael Karibian
Back cover photo by Alana Franklin

ISBN 978-1-60037-547-7

Library of Congress Control Number: 2008943938

MORGAN · JAMES
THE ENTREPRENEURIAL PUBLISHER

Morgan James Publishing, LLC
1225 Franklin Ave., STE 325
Garden City, NY 11530-1693
Toll Free 800-485-4943
www.MorganJamesPublishing.com

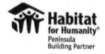

In an effort to support local communities, raise awareness and funds, Morgan James Publishing donates one percent of all book sales for the life of each book to Habitat for Humanity. Get involved today, visit **www.HelpHabitatForHumanity.org**.

Endorsements

"Wow! What a book, what an author, and what a weight loss program! If you've been carrying a belly around for a while and have been looking for a good excuse to get rid of it, *Weight Loss, Italian Style!* is that excuse. It offers a balanced, healthy, common sense approach to losing those unnecessary pounds, and you will still get to enjoy meal after meal. Please pass me the pasta. *Mangia!*"—Lewis Harrison, director of the Academy of Natural Healing, New York, and president of the International Association of Healing Professionals.

"Jill's book will change your life! I used to eat ice cream every day. Not because I wanted to. I craved it. I have not eaten ice cream in a year. The sweets craving is gone. Now I enjoy pasta, and with exercise like walking, I feel healthy, satisfied, and slim! Thank you, Jill, for my freedom from dieting!"—Anne Deidre Smith, www.HearFromYourAngels.com.

"I recommend *Weight Loss, Italian Style!* to anyone who has tried to lose weight and hasn't and to anyone who wants to learn the art of eating to live, not living to eat! The methods offered are simple and easy to maintain. I've started living like an Italian and have been dining instead of eating, moving instead of sitting, and have been breathing in nature at every opportunity. *Weight Loss, Italian Style!* will give many people freedom from diets that don't work and food that is toxic. It was a joy to read. I felt like I was in Italy and cannot wait to go!"—Karen Puma, Ventura, California.

"As a full-time 'whine expert' and occasional 'wine expert,' I highly recommend *Weight Loss, Italian Style!* It is the perfect solution for anyone who whines about losing weight but still wants to wine and dine! Jill Hendrickson's approach will make your weight loss happen, and you'll never whine again!"—January Jones, author of *Thou Shalt Not Whine ... The Eleventh Commandment.*

"At last a weight loss book that shares with the world the healthy way we eat and live on the Tuscan Isle of Elba. Jill has captured the spirit of Italian eating in a way that keeps a person well fed, deeply satisfied, and naturally slim!"—Maurizio Testa, Hotel Ilio, Isle of Elba, www.hotelilio.com.

"I can't tell you how much I enjoyed *Weight Loss, Italian Style!* It reminded me that eating is supposed to be a joyful and fulfilling experience and not something to analyze and beat myself up over. I've added pasta back into my life, and I am loving it! Finally, there's a weight loss book that's easy to understand and that brings joy back to eating, with no crazy rules."—Mary Tesch, Santa Barbara, California.

"Jill's book has great advice that really works for losing weight and keeping it off. But *Weight Loss, Italian Style!* is more than a weight loss book. It's about living a healthy life from the inside out. This is a book for your body, mind, and spirit, not about a quick, temporary fix. Plus, it's a fun read!"—Kate Phillips, life coach and financial healer, http://thegardenofplenty.com.

"It's about time somebody got the word out on how wine paired with healthy food and good companionship can actually assist the weight loss cause. The Italians have known it forever, and Jill is bringing their wisdom home to America to help Americans lose weight in the most enjoyable way possible!"—Gary Agajanian, Agajanian Vineyards, www.agajanian.com.

"Jill Hendrickson's *Weight Loss, Italian Style!* is an inspirational read for all of us struggling with weight and body image issues. (And isn't everybody?) Not the usual diet book with stringent rules by the 'food police.' I'm delighted that *Weight Loss, Italian Style!* recommends my favorite food—extra virgin olive oil—as an integral part of healthy eating. Recent studies indicate that olive oil helps to decrease one's hunger pangs, which in turn decreases your appetite and the urge to snack, all of which reinforces Jill's own experiences of dining in Italy. I'm looking forward to discovering my own *la dolce vita* and *la bella figura*!"—Nancy Ash, food consultant, owner, Strictly Olive Oil, www.strictlyoliveoil.com.

"*Weight Loss, Italian Style!* explodes the myth that pasta makes a person fat. As Jill points out, high quality pastas prepared the Italian way are an excellent choice for those who want to slim down and still eat delicious, satisfying food!"—Angelo Paolucci, president, Delverde America, Inc., www.delverde.it.

"As a person involved with fine dining for twenty-eight years, I applaud *Weight Loss, Italian Style!*'s playful attempt to wean Americans off of fattening fast food and teach them the joys of falling in love with relaxed, quality eating. This is the experience I give my guests, and it must make them happy because they keep coming back!"—Lynn Tran, Lynn's Bistro, Kirkland, Washington, www.lynnsbistro.com.

"It's no Co Winki Dink that Jill's perception and attention to detail would lead her to uncover a 'wonderful secret'—eating comfort foods AND being healthy! Sounds like a win/win for *everyone* to enjoy!"—Carrie Albright, author, grief coach, inventor, artist, Henderson, Nevada.

"Thumbs up to Jill and *Weight Loss, Italian Style!* for sharing with us the Italians' secrets to staying slender and healthy. The abundant use of extra virgin olive oil in combination with a healthy approach to life will improve the lives of all who try it!"—Kyle Sawatzky, Bari Olive Oil Company, www.barioliveoil.com.

To Mom and Dad: Thank you for always being so supportive of my passion for Italy and things Italian—and for everything else!

Acknowledgments

Thank you Dr. Barbara De Angelis for your amazing mentoring and your fierce commitment to helping me find a publishing home for *Weight Loss, Italian Style!*

Big thank-you also to David and Janet Hendrickson, John Richau, Barbara Christl, Ann Woodliff, Anne Deirdre Smith, Kate Phillips, Heidi and Mark Bonnard, Martha Debs, Robert Fries, and Loredana Lo Bianco for your love and support during the process of writing this book. Thanks, John, for emergency help with the computer and for the impromptu Italian-style parties!

Grazie mille to Rudy Ascibahian and Loredana Lo Bianco for your knowledge of the Italian language and to Rudy for technical and artistic advice related to Italian food.

Special praise goes to Debbie Feldstein for her keen eye, sharp pencil, and sharp wit, and to Jenny Hamby for her much appreciated copywriting assistance.

Many thanks to David Hancock of Morgan James Publishing and Rick Frishman of Planned TV Arts for seeing the potential of *Weight Loss, Italian Style!* and for taking a chance with it and with me.

I'd like to thank everyone in my Transformation Circle group and also Megan Washburn, Sherry Duke, Antonio Frontera, Andrea Contarin, Mike Karibian, Alana Franklin, Nick and Sam Marziliano, Corrie Woods, Carol Hendrickson, Patrick Bourrel, The Tennis Gang, Jim and Penny Price, Augusto Merlini, all of my colleagues, students, and teachers past and present, and all the others who helped me— including those who did so without even knowing it.

Finally, thank-you to Italy and the Italian people for igniting the inspiration to write *Weight Loss, Italian Style!* May you continue to honor and enjoy your extraordinary cuisine and share it with the rest of the world!

Foreword

I am Italian, (well, Italian-American) and I realized during my last trip to Italy that Italians are not fat! I had always carried around an image of Italians as being heavy and round, but to my surprise, the last time I was there, I discovered that they were all in shape and gorgeous. Many ordinary people looked like the models we see in magazines. I was wondering how this could be and realized that Jill has all the reasons in *Weight Loss, Italian Style!*

We Americans don't seem to understand that our way of life and the images we put in our minds have everything to do with the way we look. On my last visit to Italy, I, like Jill, realized how active Italians are compared to Americans. They walk everywhere or they ride their bikes. One way or another, they're always on the move.

They also know how to eat. Most of us have heard the saying, "You are what you eat," since we were kids. Well, it's true. If you eat a lot of junk, don't expect to look good, like the Italians. I recently lost a lot of weight by eating portions of protein no bigger than the size of my fist. (An Italian idea.) I also love to cook and eat pasta. I try to eat whole wheat pasta whenever I can, as it contains more nutrients than regular pasta. As Jill points out, pasta doesn't make you fat.

Many people believe that pasta will make them fat because it's made with flour. But the kind of white flour used in cookies and cakes is a different than the hard durum wheat semolina used in Italian pasta. It isn't pasta that makes people fat. It's the cream and all the other bad stuff we Americans add to pasta that makes us put on the pounds. Plus, we eat too much of it at one sitting. That's not the Italian way.

So, don't underestimate carbs. They're necessary for the proper functioning of our bodies. We need energy, and carbs provide it for us. Learn to love your carbs, but in the right way—the Italian way.

I also believe, as Jill does, that the mind is an underused tool in weight loss. We wonder why thin people don't put on weight. One reason is that they believe they are thin and, consequently, act the part. So thinness is what they achieve. It all starts with the mind and knowing how to use it.

Lastly, the clean, wholesome food that people eat in Italy is something we are missing here in America. When I was in Italy, we actually milked our cow to get milk. We didn't buy it at the store. Italian food is fresh, without all the chemicals we are accustomed to eating. There are no chemicals in most of their foods. I side with the Italians on this and feel that avoiding processed foods and eating organically can be a big factor in weight loss.

So, as you visit Italy through Jill's wonderful and en*light*ening book, understand that the fact that Italians live *La Dolce Vita* and look thin and gorgeous is greatly due to the way they eat and their active lifestyle. Put it in your mind that you can have this, too. Then go out and achieve it and enjoy the beautiful life that God has given you.

— Chef Antonio Frontera, author,

Chicken Soup for the Soul Kids in the Kitchen:
Tasty Recipes and Fun Activities for Budding Chefs

Contents

Introduction

Welcome, and thank you for purchasing this book. It's my sincere hope that my story of lasting weight loss will inspire you and motivate you to achieve what I've done. And I know you can do it, too!

How can I be so sure that success is waiting for you? After all, I don't know you. But here's something I *do* know: unlike millions of people who are stuck in the misery of being overweight, you've decided to take action. Rather than allowing your weight to control your life, you're on a mission to control your weight. And when you decided to purchase this book, you took the first step.

So welcome, thank you, and congratulations! You're on the way to a whole new you and a whole new way of life.

Why You're Here

I know why you're here. You're embarrassed to wear shorts. When you go to a party you look around to see if you're the largest person in the room. You've tried everything—exercising until you drop, plus every diet that ever came down the pipeline. And nothing works. A problem looms large in your life, and you're down on yourself for failing to deal with it. You probably mistakenly believe that if you want to achieve a healthy size you're going to have to give up tasty foods for the rest of your life.

With those negative thoughts, it's no wonder that like the other two-thirds of Americans who are overweight, you find the idea of a diet as unappetizing as steamed brussels sprouts. (Nothing against brussels sprouts!)

But what if there were a safe and enjoyable way of losing weight and keeping it off? What if there were a lifestyle approach you could take that could eliminate the stress, aggravation, and futility of dieting? What if this method actually encouraged you to eat "forbidden" foods such as pizza and pasta? What if it increased your sensual enjoyment of eating and, therefore, overall life?

I bet those negative thoughts above would vanish in an instant.

Well, get ready to get positive—and positively svelte! The method exists. *Weight Loss, Italian Style! Ditch the Diet, Pass the Pasta, and Drop the Pounds FOREVER* gives you an insider's look at how millions of Italians keep weight off without even thinking about it. That's why you rarely see obese people in Italy. Not in Rome, not in Florence, not in Venice. Not at the airport, on the trains, or at the beach—unless they're tourists.

How this "Diet" Was Born

I've traveled the world, from Istanbul to India, from one side of the United States to the other. And almost everywhere I went, people had a love-hate relationship with eating. They loved food but hated the weight they gained when they indulged in favorite foods. When I traveled to Italy, however, I discovered a country full of vibrant people who adore food without shame, regret, or a major problem with the scales! When Italians are hungry, they eat, and they eat with gusto. Yet despite a diet rich in pasta, cheese, and other things that you may think of as diet no-no's, Italians don't have nearly the weight problem we experience in the States.

The more I saw, the more I wanted to know their secret.

Get Ready to Reprogram Your Thinking

The American idea that Italian food makes you fat is *wrong*. I've lived in Italy, and you couldn't prove it by me or by the Italians. They're not only much trimmer than Americans, they're among the slimmest people in all of Europe, according to European Commission findings—despite the fact that they can't live without their pizza, pasta, and gelato.

While Americans continue to fight a never-ending battle against the bulge, Italians go about eating a delicious and satisfying diet that includes many of your favorite forbidden foods. Most don't diet as we know it. Unlike Americans, traditional Italians know how to eat for maximum pleasure and minimum damage to their figures. How can this be possible in a country with arguably the best food on the planet? A country where eating takes center stage in all of family and social life? Where it provides such a major source of pleasure that it could be described as the national pastime? Their secret is the one I learned through my own experience. And the best part is, you don't have to go all the way to Italy, the way I did, to learn and apply the method. The principles are so simple you can practice them here at home. And I'll share them with you in a conversational, readable style that I hope you'll enjoy in the pages to come.

I'll show you how Italians break all the so-called diet rules that have been making you miserable—and which can actually sabotage your ability to lose weight. They enjoy bread and cheese and four- or five-course meals. They drink wine. They wouldn't dream of stooping to low-fat, no-fat "fake" versions of food. And they love their carbs.

It's not a pipe dream to imagine yourself slimming down and keeping the weight off while still enjoying all your favorite foods. It's a dream come true! It happens all the time to American women who go to Italy to live and study. Many end up not only with a new body of knowledge about an amazing culture, but also with new and more attractive physical bodies—plus altered attitudes about eating and exercise that help them keep the weight off for the rest of their lives. And all you have to do is follow the habits of smart Italians: to eat and eat well.

What You'll Learn

Weight Loss, Italian Style! invites you to ditch your self-defeating diet mentality and replace it with a joyful love affair with food. To get you started, I'll tell you about my close encounter with *La Dolce Vita.* You'll share my surprise at losing weight while eating my way through Tuscany, where the natives rank the enjoyment of food among life's most worthy pleasures. (Tuscans are my kind of people!)

Let's face it. Lugging around extra weight isn't fun. Neither is starving yourself. Loving food, looking forward to delicious meals without having to worry about packing on the pounds—now that's what I call living.

In *Weight Loss, Italian Style!* you'll learn how to lose weight in a natural way that increases your zest for life because you feel great and enjoy everything life has to offer, including great food. I'll tell you just how easy it is to prepare delicious meals and create an entire Italian dining experience, whether you love to cook or whether you hate it. (And to prove it, I've created a special recipe collection for you to download from my website at www.WeightLossItalianStyle.com/bonus.)

So, *carpe diem*—seize the day! (Or, in this case, seize *Weight Loss, Italian Style!*) There really is a better way. You *can* master your eating habits by taking inspiration from the world's greatest food lovers, the Italians. You *can* achieve your ideal body weight and maintain it by counting your blessings instead of your calories.

The Italians, who combine passion and sensitivity in the preparation of food, taught the French a thing or two about cooking. Following their example, *Weight Loss, Italian Style!* will teach you how to eat in a way that lets you ditch the diet, pass the pasta, and drop the pounds—forever.

Now that's what I call *La Dolce Vita* in any language!

Chapter 1:

The Accidental Diet

Let me set the stage for you. I was packing for my dream trip to Italy. It was supposed to be my break for fun and relaxation before returning to face the singles scene again after three years of a grueling divorce. Just before I zipped my suitcase shut, I remembered that I needed to pack my bathing suit, which I hadn't worn in a while since there aren't many swimming opportunities in Manhattan. I pulled it on and went to the mirror. I was happy with what I saw until I turned and caught a glimpse of my backside in the reflection.

Oh, my God! Where did *that* come from? My rear end seemed to have settled south, and there were two saddlebags of fat dripping from the place where my buttocks used to meet my thighs. When had the trim, taut figure of my youth turned into *this?* I'd just turned forty and knew I'd put on a couple of pounds while sitting at my desk, banging out my master's thesis. But *this* came as a shock.

Then I was hit with another terrifying thought. If I looked like this now, what was I going to look like when I got back from the land of pizza and pasta? Surely I would come home looking like a blimp—only wider. I was devastated. But with my trip looming so close, there was no time to do anything about it. In despair, I almost left the swimsuit behind. But at the last minute, I tossed it in my suitcase. I'm glad that I did.

Flash forward. It's ten years later, and you know what? I still have that bathing suit. No, it's not a moth-eaten souvenir that I keep tucked away in my memory box. It still fits. Because unbeknownst to me, while I was headed for the right place to buy a great pair of stylish shoes or pay a visit to Trevi Fountain, I was also about to discover a lifestyle approach to eating that has keep me slim for more than a decade.

Seen on the *Via Veneto*

A funny thing happened on the way to the Forum. I hadn't been there in years, and what struck me as I walked through the streets of Rome was how trim the Italians looked compared to their counterparts in America. Yet there they were, eating pizza and pasta at outdoor restaurants and lining up for gelatos.

When in Rome, they say, do as the Romans. And did I ever! I couldn't resist the food and didn't even try. In fact, I spent most of my vacation casting caution to the wind and breaking every diet rule known to mankind. I drank lattes for breakfast, ate pizzas for lunch, and indulged in four-course dinners. I had gelatos, drank wine, and enjoyed some glorious desserts. Calisthenics? No chance. The closest thing I engaged in was bending my elbow to spoon another delicious scoop of tiramisu into my mouth!

You probably won't be surprised when I tell you that halfway through my trip, the elastic in my pants gave out. But I'll bet this next revelation will shock you. As I was wondering where I was going to buy another pair of pants to fit my expanded abdomen, I glanced into the mirror and saw to my astonishment that the problem wasn't that the elastic had stretched out. My waist had stretched in! The pants were hanging on my hips instead of sitting at my waist because I'd lost weight. My stomach had shrunk! But how was it possible with all that eating? I was astounded and skeptical that I would ever be able to maintain that once I got home.

I'll bet *you're* skeptical, too. That's okay. Be skeptical. Just don't stop reading.

Italian Style in America

I know what you're thinking. "How nice for you, Jill. But I'm not planning on crossing the Atlantic anytime soon. So how I can possibly lose weight Italian style?" That's a good question. And I've got a good answer. My story's not over yet. Fast forward to December, the same year as my Italian getaway. I wasn't in Italy anymore; I was back in Manhattan. It wasn't warm and sunny. It was dreary and cold. And I wasn't sitting at some outdoor restaurant, sipping cappuccino. I was trudging down Broadway in the snow, looking at people bundled up to their necks looking more like overstuffed igloos than people. But I hadn't reverted into the abominable snowwoman. I was still as slim, trim, and *molto bene* as when I'd left Rome.

When I returned, I'd wanted to race right back to *la bell' Italia*, where life felt sweet and carefree, but I couldn't because I was locked in a legal battle that would keep me in Manhattan for the next few years. So I did the next best thing. I brought Italy to New York and lived like an Italian. And it saved me from middle-aged spread.

How did I recreate the Italian experience in America? *Boh!* as the Italians would say with a shrug. It wasn't that hard. And if I can do it, you can do it. Why wait? Let's get started.

Andiamo. Read on …

Island Time

For you to understand the skills and the attitude I brought back to America that have made staying slim so easy, I need to tell you what I saw and experienced in Italy. Although I'd begun my trip in Rome, I spent the majority of my time on the Isle of Elba, in Tuscany, where I studied Italian. I stayed at a small hotel with an Italian meal plan that allowed me to eat breakfast and dinner at the hotel and do whatever I wanted for lunch. Here was the routine:

I started the day with a light Italian breakfast of a cappuccino or a latte and a *cornetto* (a type of Italian croissant) and a piece of fruit. Fresh, delicious, and it was so much more satisfying than my usual humongous New York bagel slathered in butter and jam. Then I strolled down the beach to my language lessons, a thirty-minute walk. Class was held on the terrace of another hotel overlooking the ocean. We studied for a couple hours, then broke for espressos and more cappuccinos. At 1:00 PM, class finished for the day, and I'd walk back along the beach and up an incline to the hotel. Sometimes I would grab a pizza on my way home, or I'd eat a three-course afternoon meal at the hotel. No day went by without at least one plate of pasta, sometimes two. After lunch I'd study, then go sightseeing or swimming in the ocean. But I'd always be home for a four-course dinner with fellow students at 8:00 PM.

It was on this unlikely regime that my pants starting falling off of me. (Not because the men were so charming, which they were!) But how had it happened? How had I lost weight eating so much food? And more importantly, how could I take that experience with me back to America and leave the fat behind in Tuscany?

After some contemplation, I realized it boiled down to two things: the specifics of what and how I ate and the amount of unintentional exercise I was getting. Everything on Elba was fresh, fresh, fresh. We ate lots of fish and only in-season fruits and vegetables that were on the table at every meal. The food was simply prepared, which showcased rather than smothered its natural flavors. There were no heavy sauces, and I didn't eat anything with preservatives. The fresh-baked bread was so tasty that it made butter unnecessary, which was a good thing since butter was seen on the table only at breakfast. And I never used it then, because the *cornetti* tasted great without it.

Italian-style dining is luxurious. Our meals were divided into courses spread over an hour or more, so it always seemed like I was enjoying a lot of food. We drank both wine and sparkling mineral water with dinner. And there was always dessert—rich and delightful Italian custard, for example—or an overflowing basket of fruits. When the meal was over, we either gathered for coffee on the patio, played ping-pong, or went for walks. Occasionally we went out dancing.

One way or another, I was always moving, even with class four hours a day and a couple hours of studying. Just scaling the steps to Napoleon's home in the harbor city of Portoferraio winded me at first. And unlike some Italian hotels, mine had an elevator, but it was so small and inconvenient I used the stairs—four sets of them—several times a day. Sightseeing on the island required strong legs and stamina, too. But after only a couple of weeks on Elba, my glutes were harder and my strength increased, and I was carrying around less body weight to boot.

Three Square Meals a Day Don't Make You Round

What else was different about my island lifestyle? I ate three meals a day, not counting my afternoon gelato. You probably think three meals a day is normal. But tell me this: do you eat three meals a day? In my life before Tuscany, my daily food intake consisted of three meals plus whatever delectable item gave me one of those "come hither" looks from the windows along Broadway. I didn't have willpower and never even bothered trying to resist any goodies because one, I was always hungry, and two, well, because they were there! (I admit it. I was a habitual snacker.)

That was then. This is now. After my time in Italy, I vowed that I would change my relationship to food. And, you know what? I did. On the sleepy little Isle of Elba, I learned to kick the Great American Diet Downfall (between-meal snacking) by discovering the biggest secret to life-long weight loss and maintenance: Eat like an Italian. In other words, eat well at every meal. Then you won't be hungry in between. Wow, what a concept.

Now you might be wondering exactly how an educated woman in the twenty-first century could make it to the age of forty without knowing the value of eating well at meals. But I have a feeling that there are a lot more people out there who are just as clueless as I was. You know why I think that? According to the Centers for Disease Control and Prevention:

At least two-thirds of US adults, or 66 percent of the adult population, is either overweight or obese.

And the rate could be higher, since the most recent statistics were gathered a couple of years ago. Americans are fighting, but losing, the battle of the bulge.

Despite the information available on weight and health, there are a lot of "uneducated" people out there. And no wonder. Just where are we supposed to learn these good eating habits? From the commercial messages we get on television? In the aisles of the twenty-four-hour convenience stores and fast food restaurants dedicated to profits, not health?

Do we learn them from a culture that turns holidays and celebrations into unhealthy gorge-a-thons? After all, what's Thanksgiving without turkey and stuffing or a birthday without a birthday cake? Believe me; the idea of eating three of the right kind of meals a day was radical to me. It sounds ridiculously simple, but it changed my life. That is saying a lot, because I was the sweet eater to end all sweet eaters. And until my body started rebelling, I never saw anything wrong with it. Then, when I realized that I had a full-fledged sugar monkey on my back, I wasn't sure I could ever break the cycle of unhealthy eating. I figured I was a "lifer," sentenced to a never-ending battle with food where I was always the loser.

You *Can* Go Home Again

It's always darkest before the dawn. And just as things were about to go completely black, I saw the light on Elba. Eating three Italian meals a day and eating the Italian way made everything easy. Convenience foods became a thing of the past. I stopped eating them because I no longer craved them. I had become accustomed to the taste of real food. I signed up with a food co-op that dropped off fresh produce once a week at a church across the street. That caused two things to happen. One, I began cooking better things for myself instead of going out so much, which made a huge difference. It also caused me to spend less time in grocery stores, which meant less browsing through the cookie and potato chip sections—another plus.

I began eating fruit for dessert, like I did on Elba, instead of ice cream and ice cream substitutes. And I paid better attention to my portions. I ditched all that nonsense about no carbs. It really frustrates me when people in America are told they have to give up carbs and all the other things they love if they want to lose weight. I'm a living example that that isn't true. So is almost every man, woman, and child in Italy!

Love Your Carbs

What happens when you cut out carbs? You crave them, don't you? You know what I mean. You're on some awful diet and you're eating lettuce and celery sticks for lunch, but what you really want is something filling, like a piece of pizza. There you are, cutting the lettuce into tiny bites to try to make it seem as if you're eating something that makes you happy, but it doesn't work. You're unsatisfied, and you know it. So by mid-afternoon, you're raiding the freezer, digging into a gallon of ice cream—with cookies on top—cursing carbohydrates and probably beating up on yourself for your lack of will power.

Don't be so hard on yourself. You aren't the problem! Carbs aren't the problem. The problem is the way we eat and live in America. Due to our harried lifestyle and an advertising industry that pushes unhealthy food at every opportunity, we've lost all common sense when it comes to eating, exercising, and enjoying the blessing that food really is. It's time to stop the madness.

You don't have to give up your carbs. In fact, I'm going to encourage you to eat them. Why? Because Italians eat them and get by just fine. But they eat them in proper proportions. And not all day long. They eat just enough that they're not hungry until their next meal.

11

I mentioned that I ate a relatively light breakfast each morning and that my biggest meal was the one I enjoyed each evening. It's the complete opposite of what the so-called, self-proclaimed diet gurus recommend. They say you're supposed to load up on calories in the morning and that breakfast is the most important meal of the day. The most important meal for whom? The fast food franchises? The pancake pushers? It's not the most important meal for me, and certainly not for the Italians.

The Meal That Lives Up to Its Name

Traditionally Italians have never eaten much breakfast—just a roll or a couple of cookies and what for us would be a rather small cup of coffee. (Think Stella D'oro Breakfast Treats.) That's it, although some are eating cereal nowadays. No, Italians take a light approach to breakfast and save their calories for the more sumptuous fare at lunch and dinner. And you know what? It isn't killing them or fattening them up. They're slimmer and healthier than most Americans. They must be doing something right!

If you ask Italians why they eat so little for breakfast, they'll shrug. Most don't even think about it. My guess is that they eat so well at night they're not that hungry in the morning. And think about this: does the human body really *need* a lot of food first thing in the morning after it's been asleep for eight hours? When the alarm clock goes off, your organs are not oiled and running, and you're hardly even awake. That doesn't sound like the time for a big calorie extravaganza to me. Does it to you?

The morning meal is called "breakfast" for a reason. You're breaking a fast. You've had nothing in your stomach for eight to twelve hours, maybe more. And as anyone knows, you don't break a fast by gorging. Your digestive system can't take the onslaught. When you recommence eating after a fast, you start out small and work your way up to something more substantial later, like lunch, which hopefully is a social occasion when you get to enjoy the company of other people and make your meal more of an event.

Now, I like breakfast as much as the next person. But after my Italian experience, I've trained myself to want less of it. Why? Because there's a shorter waiting period between breakfast and lunch than between lunch and dinner, and I'd rather save the calories for things like lasagna and manicotti at the more social meals when I can linger. And while it's not a good idea to go to bed directly after dining heavily, it is true that what you eat for dinner has to last you until dawn. So, it stands to reason that you might want something more for your last meal of the day, especially if you eat in the early evening, than for your first meal.

Your Weight in Balance

Changing my breakfast habit was just the beginning of a new and carefree way of living and eating that has made staying slim almost effortless. The other part of the equation is exercise, or perhaps I should say an active lifestyle, because I'm not really talking about going to the gym. When I got back from Italy, I realized that being active had to be part of the fabric of my daily life just as much as eating was. My goal became to move as much as possible at every opportunity. I started walking more around Manhattan instead of *always* taking buses, subways, and taxis. I even walked up the stairs to my apartment occasionally instead of using the elevator. (I say "occasionally" because I lived on the fourteenth floor, and a marathon climbing session wasn't always possible.)

The Italian way of life became integrated into *my* way of life. I learned that body, mind, and spirit all need to be working in unison for the "accidental diet" to stick. We'll be talking more about this in the rest of the book, but for now, think of it this way: a bird needs two wings and a tail to fly. So does an airplane. You, too, need this kind of balance in order to lift yourself out of your weight-based blues and soar. If you haven't succeeded in losing weight in the past, it's almost a given that you were out of balance in one, if not all three, of these areas.

But don't worry. With my help you can learn how to master eating, moving, and managing your mind for healthy weight loss and carefree maintenance. And you know what? Once you've mastered your mind, you'll find that eating and moving fall naturally into place. Why? Because your mind is the master of your life. When your inner world is handled, the outside takes care of itself. Sound too good to be true? Let me assure you, it's not going to be that difficult. It wasn't for me.

In fact, it was a relief to find a strategy for eating and living, because having a plan to follow makes things simple.

Don't Follow the Rules—Break Them!

Italians don't like rules and flaunt them whenever possible. (It's one of the things I like about losing weight Italian style.) So I'm not going to crush you or your spirit with a bunch of rigid rules to follow. Instead, I'm going to offer you some practical, pleasant suggestions for how to live and eat better and more like an Italian in order to look and feel like one—in other words, sexy, vivacious, and healthy, healthy, healthy.

So, *benvenuta!* I invite you to let me show you how to live in a way that allows you to eat good food and still lose weight—or just maintain it. I know that sounds like a pretty tall order. How are we going to manage it? The same way the Romans pulled off a minor miracle by creating one of the largest, most enduring empires in world history. We're going to break it down into pieces using Caesar's war strategy:

Divide and Conquer!

Chapter 2:

The Body-Mind Connection and *La Bella Figura*

I saw the angel in the marble and carved until I set him free.
—Michelangelo

While the ancient Romans grew their empire by dividing and conquering, they maintained it and kept the peace by partnering with former enemies when possible. Likewise, if you want to lose weight, it makes sense to befriend your body and enlist its cooperation rather than fight against it.

What is your attitude toward your body? Are you at war with it, or are you at peace? Really think about it. If you're not happy with it, you're pitting yourself against yourself, which creates a no-win situation. Because the truth is, your body is benign; it simply follows orders. It takes what it's given and does the best it can with what it gets. What does this mean to you? If you've been feeding your body a steady diet of junk food, you shouldn't be surprised with the results. As a friend of mine says, "If you plant corn, don't expect rutabagas." So before we do anything else, it's important to consider your relationship with your physical being.

Your body is what you've made it. If you want it to change, you've got to treat it better. Be honest with yourself about the ways you may be abusing it, then make a conscious effort to stop. Think kindly toward your physical being, no matter what state it's in right now. Many people treat their cars better than they treat themselves. But if your body breaks down—which it eventually will if you feed it incorrectly—the consequences are a lot worse than if your car goes into the shop. Still, with loving care, your body can be transformed and restored to its natural, healthy state.

Mind Games

There's probably more than an ounce of truth to the joke that when women look at themselves in the mirror they see faults, but when men look at themselves, they see God's gift to women. So right now, before you do anything else, take this book with you and go to a full-length mirror, if you have one, and look at yourself. (If you don't have a full-length mirror, think about investing in an inexpensive one. It's important to be able to see what you look like—*really* look like.)

As you stand before the mirror, give yourself the once-over. Then observe different parts of your body. Ask yourself these questions:

- **What am I feeling about what I see?** (If you're nowhere near a mirror, then close your eyes and imagine going to a mirror and looking at your reflection.)
- **What words and thoughts come to me when I view my image?** If you're like a lot of women, you may feel more critical than loving.
- **Am I comfortable with what I see?**
- **Does my energy sink at the sight of myself, or do I feel uplifted?**

- **Do I view my physical self as an adversary or a friend?** Are you pleased with your reflection, or does your inner critic chime in?

Women have been conditioned to feel imperfect so that others, including the advertising industry, can manipulate us. It's not right and it's not fair, but it takes an incredible amount of self-esteem to counteract the negative messages we're bombarded with each day. Please! If you want your body's cooperation with your weight loss efforts, ignore what the media tells you about female standards of beauty, and work on self-acceptance. This is crucial to your long-term success. Why? Because a critical attitude toward yourself or your body creates a resistance that makes it harder to lose weight.

Think of how you respond internally when someone criticizes you. Do you want to cooperate with them, or do you want to fight back? Think how people respond when *you* criticize *them*. Does it ever work? Does it achieve the result you're seeking? Probably not. Bees respond better to honey than salt. People respond better to words of encouragement than blame.

I Love You Just the Way You Are

Your body responds better to self-love than self-loathing. After all, your body is simply an extension of yourself. And you don't hate yourself, do you? You shouldn't. You're a perfect human exactly as you are. Your body size, shape, or type doesn't affect that. What it does affect is your health and well-being.

There's nothing wrong with you unless you're so overweight that it poses a health risk, and even then it's something to be treated with compassion rather than contempt. Can you just hold lightly in your mind some modifications you'd like to make while thinking well of yourself however you are? Your body is more malleable than you imagine and responds even to your thoughts. In fact, while the brain is confined to your head, your mind pervades your entire body. You're in communication with every cell at all times, so be careful about the messages you send.

The deep-seated meanness many of us feel toward ourselves causes us to wall off entire parts of ourselves and reject them. We may not even be aware that we do this. Part of the process of retrieving your life and overcoming your weight issues involves reawaking and embracing the rejected parts. Because it's the things you reject and neglect that ultimately rule you by popping up and derailing you at the least convenient times. For example, have you ever known someone who has tried repeatedly to lose weight but who always manages to sabotage their efforts just before they reach their goal? It's unconscious, but they possess a self-defeating element that they haven't addressed.

The Real Reason to Lose Weight Italian Style

I need to ask you something. Just why are you interested in losing weight? It's a legitimate question. Is it because you care about your health and want to be the healthiest person possible? Or is it because you think you need to fit someone else's standard of beauty? Before you travel any further on your weight loss path, now is the time to ask yourself:

- Where did I get my ideas about what's beautiful?
- Can I appreciate my own beauty regardless of how much I weigh?
- Do I withhold self-approval based on my weight?
- On what do I base my judgments about my body?
- Are my criteria even valid?

There are no right or wrong answers. It's all just food—for thought!

You Are the Eye of the Beholder

If you look at the way the female form has been depicted throughout history—in sculpture and paintings, say—you'll see some very full figures, including some that nowadays would be considered downright hefty. There was actually a time in Italy when it was a compliment to call somebody fat, because it meant they had enough money to eat well. Rent a copy of Fellini's *La Dolce Vita*. In it, Anita Ekberg is no toothpick. She's a voluptuous 1950s-style beauty who would today be considered fat. Yet hardly anyone would argue with the fact that in the Trevi Fountain scene, she looks like Venus rising from the sea.

I can think of a lot of famous women who are full figured and are considered beautiful. Queen Latifah, Jennifer Hudson, and even the Venus de Milo come to mind. When I see their pictures, I never think that they'd be more beautiful if they were thin. They look great the way they are. So I urge you to let your desire to lose weight be about your health first and foremost, not about how many pounds you want to weigh or what dress size you think you should wear—and certainly not to please anybody else.

We women fill too many of our waking hours attempting to attain standards of beauty that are illusive and then beating ourselves up for failing to attain those standards. Wouldn't it be nice to just relax and not have to worry about it? To just feel accepted and to love yourself the way you are? (I'm not talking about egotistical love. I'm talking about a healthy self-respect. There's a big difference.) Can you take a break from the relentless quest for perfection for the rest of the day? More important than how you look on the outside is how you feel within, because the inside impacts the outside, probably more than anything else. The real work with weight loss and maintenance starts and ends with your inner state.

You don't have to be thin to be beautiful. The only person you need to please is you. Beauty is so subjective. Standards vary from culture to culture and change over time. I think back to when I was in my thirties, in a demoralizing marriage, and being criticized on a regular basis. By societal standards, I was probably better looking then than I am now, but I prefer myself now, because I like myself better.

Back then I was being disparaged by the person closest to me, so when I looked in the mirror, all I saw were my faults. What on earth were they? I can't even remember. They may have multiplied exponentially with age, but I no longer judge myself that way. I'm thankful for what I've got. And I wish the same for you. And here's something that may really shock you: you may even find you don't have a weight problem once your self-image gets upgraded.

La Bella Figura

The Italians place a lot of importance on *la bella figura*—even more than we do. The literal translation is "the beautiful figure," but the *meaning* is closer to "cutting a good image" or "looking good." It has to do with appearance, yes, but not simply weight and curves. It refers to a person's way of presenting themselves, their behavior, and aesthetics in general.

The funny thing is that most Italians think they cut a *bella figura* even when they don't, which can be quite comical to outsiders. (For a glimpse of this, see some of the movies of comedic actor Roberto Benigni.) The Italian attitude is instructive. We can learn from it! You see, in a certain sense, *la bella figura* depends as much on how you think of yourself as on how you look. How is that possible? It's because others tend to mirror back your attitude toward yourself, and because in a very real sense, it's only what *you* think that matters.

Instead of looks, let's talk about power. You've probably met some pretty unprepossessing people who are able to command a lot of respect simply by the way they carry themselves. You've probably also met people of great power who undercut their authority by presenting themselves in a meek or retiring way. By the same token, no matter how good looking you are, if you don't feel it on the inside and project those feelings you're not going to impact the world much. People will pick up on your lack of self-esteem.

Love Thyself

There are many people in our lives whose opinions we care about, but the most important relationship you have is with yourself. It's crucial that you feel good about yourself and understand that if you never change another thing about yourself, you're still perfect. What makes you perfect is your individuality. There's no one like you on the face of the earth. You're one-of-a-kind … singular. And don't ever forget it!

In a world where others will to try to take you down, including those closest to you, your best safety net is a healthy self-concept. So, come on. Do you think you're beautiful? Do you *treat* yourself as if you're beautiful? Studies show that 29 percent of Italian women are unhappy with their bodies, so you're clearly not alone if you think you're flawed. In fact, a report published by the YWCA in August 2008 titled, "Beauty at Any Cost," suggests from a variety of statistics that a whopping 80 percent of women are unhappy with the way they look. The study concludes that an obsession with an unattainable appearance fostered by the diet, fashion, and cosmetics industries creates a lifelong burden for women, including serious health and even financial consequences.

Are any of us surprised? No. Are any of us victims? Yes. Far too many women (and men) allow their negative self-images to rob them of a full life. Let's make sure you're not one of them! Keep reading …

Ugly Duckling Syndrome

I grew up feeling like an ugly duckling, or at least a plain Jane. My face started breaking out when I was ten. I had a surgical scar across my lower abdomen that my bathing suit bottom barely covered. I had big feet and an older sister who was prettier. I thought I could find salvation in the advice of women's magazines, but they only made things worse.

Like many young girls, I started reading those magazines when I was eleven or twelve because they promised solutions to every beauty problem under the sun and gave me a window to the world of adults. But those magazines gave me and every adolescent girl I knew (not to mention the grown-up women) something new to worry about on top of everything else in life. The magazines were overwhelmingly filled with articles about dieting. They made it clear that I and every other reader probably had a weight problem and that we'd better do something about it.

This is how even as young girls we begin to assess ourselves negatively and develop distorted ideas of how we should eat and look due to unhealthy messages from the media. But worse than what we hear or see is what we do to ourselves because of it. We magnify the negative messages a hundred times in our minds. Think of some negative comment someone once made about you … and shame on them for saying it. But what did you do with it? Rather than reject the message, you probably repeated it to yourself for the rest of the day, if not for the rest of your life.

I'd never even thought about my weight until I started reading those magazines. But once I *did* start, the worries and self-doubt began. If I didn't eat the way they suggested, was I going to become fat? Was I fat already? I remember reading once that I was only supposed to eat lettuce with half of a cling peach with a dollop of cottage cheese and a hamburger patty for lunch. I understood those articles to mean that I shouldn't be eating the way I liked, that there was something wrong with enjoying food, and worse yet, that there was something wrong with me.

As I began to fill out toward the age of fourteen, my tummy started rounding along with my thighs, and I started worrying about the broadening of my backside because of a comment someone made. I imagined this was the beginning of "becoming fat," and I was terrified because I was just starting to grow up. I remember trying the meal replacement drinks that were coming on the market at that time and also trying to follow the so-called "meal plans of the stars" that were the bread-and-butter of fashion magazines. (Fortunately, since then, many magazines have adopted a more girl-power approach to health and diet.)

But back then, I just did what I was told. I tried to follow the instructions, but they didn't make sense to me because I was always hungry. The portions never satisfied me for long, and after one of those so-called meals, it wasn't long before I'd be raiding the cupboards looking for something to fill me up.

Needless to say, I didn't pick a carrot to satisfy my cravings. Like you, perhaps, I usually chose junk food loaded with sugar. And then my gut would swell and I'd feel fat. My bad feelings would make me eat more, leading to more bad feelings. I felt caught in a vicious cycle, and, in fact, I was. I was constantly ravenous, as so many growing teenagers are, but I was totally confused about how to eat right and not balloon out of my jeans. So sometimes I starved myself, and sometimes I gorged.

It was an unhealthy pattern that I never quite licked until my trip to Tuscany, when the Italians finally showed me how to nourish myself in a way that made sense.

Be Your Own Best Friend

Because of our natural tendency to magnify the worst and turn a careless comment into an overwhelming criticism, no one is as hard on us as we are on ourselves. We convince ourselves that our flaws are all people see in us. Truth be told, most people are too concerned with their own self-image to worry about yours. The good news is that we have the power to turn down the volume on our self-criticism, which is a real boon if you want to lose weight, because the criticism backfires. The first step is just becoming aware of how often you take a swipe at yourself. Then you can start applying the brakes.

This critical voice that lives in our head comes from a warped notion that we can only achieve our goals by being hard on ourselves. But it doesn't work that way. Instead of being motivational and inspirational, self-criticism *creates resistance* to necessary changes. Encouragement overcomes obstacles...another Italian idea. Remember how the Romans limited unrest by working with conquered peoples when they could rather than squelching them? They knew that too much harshness leads to rebellion.

No doubt you've encountered this in your weight loss efforts. If you're too strict and cut out everything tasty from your diet, you may be able to go with the flow for a while. Sooner or later, however, you're likely to relapse and go into a feeding frenzy. Then, if you beat yourself up for overeating, you're likely to gorge some more.

You're Dorothy *and* the Witch …

One of my favorite movies is *The Wizard of Oz*, because it so beautifully portrays the inner battle we have with ourselves. If you remember, at the end of the movie, it's revealed that the entire adventure occurred within a dream. It all took place inside Dorothy's head! There's a reason for that. It's because it's the human condition. The witch in the movie represents a suppressed part of Dorothy herself. And it's tied up with her power. As with us, when we fail to deal with certain parts of ourselves, they come up anyway and initiate a crisis. Dorothy goes on her inner journey in order to deal with her inner demons, and to remember herself—to "re-member" the broken parts and make herself whole again. It's really a story about the journey to becoming integrated.

Quieting your inner critic has the same effect as throwing water on the witch. Like Dorothy, we're all wearing the ruby slippers, but we can't find our way home—or access our real power and overcome our issues—until we silence the witch and listen to the wizard. Throwing water on the witch means seeing her for who she really is, a disowned part of ourselves that wants to be healed. You silence the witch through gradually realizing your self-worth. On the surface you may think you already have that, but if you're abusing yourself with food, that's an indication that you don't and that you need work in that area. Most people don't want to face their inner witch. But acknowledging her and dealing with her has the power to free you.

You can start dealing with her right now by focusing on what's right about you rather than what's wrong—by focusing on your beauty rather than your perceived defects. Your experience follows your attention, so if you dwell on your weight and food issues, you bring about more of what you don't want. Where's your attention? On being overweight or on being beautiful and healthy? It's time to visualize yourself the way you want to be. First create the picture, then step into it and start acting the part.

Remember what I said about Italians and *la bella figura*. Celebrate your body whatever state it's in. It's your vehicle for getting through

24

this lifetime. If you treat it like a treasure rather than a burden, it's more likely to respond in a positive way. Your weight problem is simply one of imbalance. What you're seeking is a state of equilibrium, and when you find it, you won't have to struggle.

To maintain balance in your mind, begin to detach from seeing yourself as fat. From now on you're just you, with no judgment attached. You're fine the way you are, and you don't need to change unless you want to. Losing weight isn't something you need to do in order to win your own approval or anyone else's. Just give yourself the approval, then get into the habit of thinking about what you want, rather than what you don't want. It's all about the impressions you make on your mind. The negative mental impressions we carry are like scars across our psyche or skips in the record that lead us back to repeat the same old patterns.

We can't erase the scars, but we can create better templates.

Give Yourself a Boost

I don't know about you, but if I were going to replace a worn out template, a no longer relevant model, or an outdated paradigm; if I were going to create a new "design for living," I'd want to create something zesty and pretty and just have fun with it. I'd want to provide it with some new clothes, maybe even an Italian motor scooter or at least some cool Italian sunglasses. Let your imagination go wild and just create a new mental image of yourself that you absolutely love.

Then start living it.

If you're like a lot of women, you've put entire parts of your life on hold until you are able to create a certain set of arbitrary circumstances. Perhaps you've decided you're not going to look for a boyfriend, start that project, develop a new career, or go on that vacation until you "lose the weight." But if you wait to achieve the "perfect" weight before you start living, you may wait forever and never live at all. It's natural to want everything tied up neatly before we step out of our comfort zone and take a risk. It's natural, but it's not going to happen. Life doesn't work that way.

All adventurers know that fortune favors the bold! You need to show you're willing to take the risk first. Start playing the role now, and losing the weight will be easier as life steps forward to meet you half way.

Permanent, lasting weight loss requires a new perspective and a new lease on life. And by the way, it is an adventure. You may not see that now, but you will when you come out of the other side of the tunnel. It's kind of scary going into it, but there's light at the other end.

So maybe you can't lose the weight right this moment or control your eating habits. That's okay. Just start with things you *can* control. Love yourself the way you are, and if you feel that you could use an update, go to your favorite makeup counter or boutique and get a facial or a makeover. The compliments you receive will boost your ego. That boost is just what you need to give you the self-confidence you require to commit to this transformational adventure.

It's time to stop worrying about your weight and start living your life. Don't put off your goals another day just because you have a few extra pounds (or even quite a few extra pounds) on your frame. Go for it—whatever "it" is. Living as though you have already achieved your ideal body can be a playful, fun, and passionate game. You'll find it very uplifting to know that the figure you want already exists within the one you have, just waiting to be released.

That's For Me!

Have you ever seen a thin, attractive woman and felt resentful toward her to the point where you're thinking "She must be anorexic," or "How can men stand women that skinny?" When you do that, you create resistance. You're putting up a wall between you and what you want—to become thinner. A better choice is to allow yourself to feel admiration. The shift to positive energy pulls toward you what you want rather than repelling it. View people you envy as treasure maps to where you'd like to go. Instead of tightening up and mentally downgrading them, relax, let go, and say to yourself with enthusiasm, "That's for me!"

I got this idea from one of my great teachers, Barbara De Angelis. So often when we see something we want or admire, we unconsciously push it away from ourselves through envy or a sense of unworthiness. The feeling of "That's for me!" helps you move beyond these limiting feelings. It pulls you out of stuck energy and into a place of openness that makes space for what you desire. It trains your mind to think in terms of what it wants instead of what it doesn't want. Try it and notice the immediate change you feel in your body and the improvement of your mood.

To further train your mind to dwell on what you want, we're going to put your subconscious to work for you. This lightens the load of struggling only with the physical aspect of weight loss. To demonstrate the power of impressions on your subconscious, I want you to make a "That's for Me!" collage.

Do not cheat yourself out of this exercise. You'll see why in a minute. Just get a bunch of magazines and start pulling out pictures that relate to how you'd like to look, including clothes you'd like to wear and places you'd like to go. What do you imagine the new you and your new life to look like? Don't think too hard while you're doing this. Just flip through the pages and rip out pictures that appeal to you, as well as words and phrases that mean something to you. You don't even need to think about why you're choosing them. Once you've got a pile of pictures, glue them onto a large piece of poster board.

Make it a fun, light experience. Enjoy being creative and artistic. When you're done, stand back and admire your artwork. Then hang it in a place where you'll see it many times throughout the day.

Take a Page from My (Collage) Book

To give you an idea of the power of this exercise I'll share with you my own experience with it.

A few years ago when I was in a creative mood, I quickly put together a collage made up of pictures of things I wanted in my life. I didn't think while I was doing it; I just poured through a few magazines and ripped out pictures I liked and pasted them to a big piece of poster board. One was of the Ponte Vecchio in Florence; another was of a woman riding behind a man on a motor scooter in Italy. I had a picture of the Roman Forum, one of an Italian food market, and a poster of parmigiano cheese from Parma. There was a picture of a couple dancing and one of a beach resort in Latin America, one of a jet flying through the sky, some giant parrots, one of the TKTS half-price ticket booth in New York City, Times Square, Palm Springs, some tropical fish, and a poster for the musical, *Mamma Mia!* There was a picture of a man and woman being romantic together, a picture of the Moulin Rouge in Paris, a gondolier in Venice, a couple frolicking in the ocean, and a picture of Morocco.

There was no rhyme or reason to what I put on my collage. I just chose pictures I liked. And then the magic started.

One by one, from the time I hung that collage on my wall, things began to happen. Within several months I was living in Florence near the Ponte Vecchio. I spent a lot of time visiting food markets, and I found myself zooming around Florence on the back of a motor scooter. I had moved my life and belongings to California by this time, and when I got back I started dancing again. My dance partner became my boyfriend. I ended up going to Palm Springs several times. We spent a vacation at a beautiful oceanfront resort in Mexico where we interacted with giant parrots and snorkeled with tropical fish. The next year I attended a conference in Manhattan, and we found ourselves on Times Square. Everything on the collage came true, right down to going to the TKTS booth to get the tickets to see *Mamma Mia!* We went to Venice; we had an apartment in Rome in walking distance from the Forum. We went to Parma. We didn't make it to Paris, but we watched the movie *Moulin Rouge* together.

Every time I look at that collage, I'm astounded by the power of focusing your intentions and feeding the mind pictures of what you want to happen in your life. Within five years, everything on that collage had come true, except for the trip to Morocco, which I guess is on the way. Either that or I'm supposed to take up belly dancing.

Or maybe it's time to make a new collage.

How could a bunch of pictures glued to a piece of poster board be so powerful? Because success starts with having a clear picture of what you want, and the pictures of what I wanted were staring me in the face every time I ate, worked on my computer, or talked on the phone. I'd sit there, unconsciously looking at them, and my mind started to play with those impressions and mold them into reality.

I guarantee that this exercise will help you, too, develop a strong mental image of what you want for yourself—one that will work even while you're sleeping. It's part of "creative visualization," and it's used by superstar athletes, business people, and anyone with a goal to achieve.

Often we can imagine a new life, but we forget to put ourselves in it, so as you're doing your collage, don't forget to put "you" in the picture. You can even cut out a photo of yourself, use a felt pen or scissors to trim yourself down a little, and stick it on a picture of someplace you'd like to visit. Stick it on a picture of Rome or Venice. Stick yourself on a gondola with a handsome gondolier poling you down the Grand Canal.

And cut out some pictures of Roman goddesses while you're at it, like Venus on the half shell. Stick them on your "That's for Me!" collage and see what happens. We women are walking representations of a collection of goddesses, so you might as well acknowledge it. If you find a picture of Botticelli's *Birth of Venus*, cut out a picture of your face and stick it on her body. I'm not kidding. Go crazy with this. It's a lot of fun.

And, not only that, it works.

So now that you've created your template, let's move things ahead even further with …

Your Action Plan—Steps You Can Take *Now*

Buy a Journal or Notebook

Just a little one you can tuck into your purse to help you monitor negative self-talk. Write down whatever mean things pop into your head and review them at the end of the day. Would you talk to someone you liked that way? Does anyone deserve to have their self-esteem attacked? (No!)

Have I done this exercise? ___Yes ___No

If yes, jot down the benefits here. If no, write the reason:

Get a Snapper

Wear a loose-fitting rubber band on you wrist so you can "snap yourself out of it" every time you catch yourself slipping into critical self-talk. As you begin to associate mean thoughts with the painful snap, you will start training your mind to focus on the positive.

Have I done this exercise? ___Yes ___No

If yes, jot down the benefits here. If no, write the reason:

Write Your Story

During the next couple of weeks, spend five minutes a day writing in your journal about the life and the body you want. Write down what you're doing to achieve both. Then close your eyes and spend a couple minutes visualizing the new you in your new life. (See yourself not as you are but as you wish to be.)

Have I done this exercise? ___Yes ___No

If yes, jot down the benefits here. If no, write the reason:

Chapter 3:

A Love Affair (vs. a Fling)—with Food

Thou shouldst eat to live, not live to eat.
—Cicero

What is it that allows Italians from Julius Caesar to Gina Lollobrigida to keep their weight down despite having one of the most enticing cuisines on the planet? While genetics may play a part in it all, one factor is certainly their healthy respect for food. Another is their disciplined attitude towards eating, two things sorely missing from the American mindset.

Food isn't "fuel" in Italy. It's more than just sustenance. Food is a major source of pleasure for Italians. They long for it, talk about it, lovingly prepare it, savor it, and eat it with gusto. They probably even dream about it. And yet Italians are not fat.

Un Amore Appassionato

How can this be possible? It's because Italians don't treat their relationship with food as though it were a meaningless crush or passing infatuation. Not at all. Italians treat food like *un amore appassionato*, a passionate love affair. Italians make a "date" with their meals. What Americans sometimes dismiss as "feeding times" are cherished rituals to the Italians—mini celebrations, even—culminating in a deep sense of satisfaction, not unlike a long, languorous session of lovemaking. Eating Italian style leaves a person fully sated, with little desire for anything else, least of all the desire to snack.

Contrast this with the American attitude, which is more like a quickie or a one-night stand. Italians respect food. Americans lust after it. The Italian way is better for the figure. (As for which is the better approach to romance …you'll have to decide *that* for yourself!)

We live in an instant gratification society, with a fast food, microwaves, and "meal-in-a-minute" mentality that encourages us not to wait for anything. Unlike us, Italians *love* to spend quality time eating and make it a social occasion whenever possible. Their meals are sumptuous and satisfying, prepared with love and only the finest ingredients. Italians don't just eat, they *dine*. And they dine well. Do they ever!

When I travel to different places in Italy, one of the first things people ask me is, "Did you eat well?" Most of them want to know what was on my plate, but that's only a narrow sliver of eating well in Italy. For Romans, Sicilians, Milanese, and Italians from north to south, it's not just about the food. Eating is a complete sensual and emotional experience with important social implications. Food preparation and meals are intimately entwined with a sense of community and belonging. People eat with their families. Even students away from home cook and eat together. Breaking bread is a reassuring ritual that fortifies relationships. It starts and ends the day on a high note. It brings loved ones together with wine (not at breakfast!) and conversation and just the right amount of wholesome, delicious food eaten over just the right amount of time for proper digestion to take place. You leave the table physically and emotionally satisfied but never stuffed.

It sounds wonderful, and it *is* wonderful. When you allow yourself to fall in love with food again, it will mean exchanging a masochistic relationship with unhealthy eating habits for a deeply satisfying relationship with healthful food that supports your weight loss efforts. Passionate, Italian-style eating gives you a nourishing alternative to mindless gorging, inhaling fast food, or stuffing yourself in front of the TV. Eating like an Italian means learning to nurture yourself and connect with others by sharing and appreciating the blessing that food really is.

A History of Respect

On the surface, it may seem as if the obesity epidemic in the United States just underscores how much we Americans love food. But wanting to eat all the time isn't the same as loving food. When you love something—whether it's a person, a piece of priceless porcelain, or your daily meal—you show it respect. You take care of it and take time with it. There's a big difference between food adoration and gluttonous desire. The first grants slenderness, the other obesity. To illustrate: imagine the satisfaction you feel after eating a perfect chocolate truffle from a high-end chocolatier, made with all the richest, most delicious ingredients. Now imagine eating a pint of fat-free ice cream and following it up with a box of fat-free cookies. Not very satisfying, is it?

Americans have gotten this one wrong. The Italians have it right. They take food and the art of eating seriously. They eat less than we do, yet they seem to eat more, and what they eat they enjoy more than we do. It seems like a paradox, but it's not.

One of the surprising discoveries I made in Italy that radically changed my entire perspective on eating involved a simple, but shocking concept. I learned that

Your enjoyment of food exists in inverse proportion to how much you eat.

What a revelation. Shall I say it again? *The less you eat, the more you enjoy it*, and vice versa. If you never feel satisfied, it's because you're eating too much—pay attention now—of the wrong sort of things and not enough of the right sort of things (like fettuccine primavera, or pizza margherita). As a consequence, you're not extracting the greatest possible pleasure from your food.

It's no exaggeration to say that I learned how to eat in Italy. What I mean is that I learned how to temper my appetite and enjoy my food to the fullest. You can learn to do that too.

Abbondanza

Abbondanza is a word Italians use to describe plenty, like a table overflowing with food. For most of our history, America has been the land of *abbondanza*. Until recently, food was so cheap that we got into the habit of confusing abundance with overindulgence. And that's putting it mildly. Brand Steakhouse in Las Vegas, for example, will give you their 120-ounce steak (that's seven-and-a-half pounds of cow) for free if you eat the whole thing by yourself. Otherwise, you'll have to pony up $267. And Denny's Beer Barrel Pub in Pennsylvania offers their own two-, three-, and six-pound "challenge" burgers, plus a fifteen-pounder known as the "Belly Buster." (Whether the rules include a time limit or puke allowance is unknown.)

As Americans we're proud that we can afford to pile our plates high and even leave some behind if we want to, but we never do.

Gorging is a national pastime. We devote entire holidays to it. We have contests to see who can eat the most pie or corn dogs in a minute. Magazines abound with articles on how to avoid gaining pounds around the holidays, as if it's a foregone conclusion that no one can control themselves. And then it becomes a self-fulfilling prophesy.

Italy's history is different. Despite its reputation for the good life, *la bell' Italia* hasn't always been able to provide its people with enough to eat. And I'm not just talking about a distant past when most lived at a subsistence level as peasants. It was only in the second half of the twentieth century that Italy was able to overcome a long history of food insecurity.

There are Italians who can still remember suffering from food shortages as recently as World War II. Even Sophia Loren has written about her family's impoverished pantry at a time when bombs were exploding near her childhood home outside Naples. Things are different now, but plenty of Italians don't take food for granted. They respect it for its life-sustaining powers and are less willing to waste or abuse it than we are. They are also much more attuned to the subtle pleasures of eating.

In an illuminating book, *Around the Tuscan Table: Food, Family, and Gender in Twentieth-Century Florence*, Carole M. Counihan describes how the older Italians she interviewed frowned on the idea of gorging because it deadened their sense of contentment. For them, food was a source of sensual pleasure that overeating killed. They knew the secret that eludes most American "grazers":

Hunger is the best spice.

These people exercised restraint—not to torture themselves but to heighten their enjoyment! This is en*light*ened eating. They loved food so much that they weren't about to deny themselves the exquisite pleasure of having their hunger satisfied by overtaxing their taste buds.

Counihan sums up this attitude in a Florentine's saying, *poco, ma buono,* which translates loosely into, "Just a little, but make it good." You can still find this attitude among discriminating Italians, who prefer a smaller amount of high-quality food to a large amount of something inferior but less satisfying. Choosing quality over quantity and respecting that quality is the key to the art of eating well and to losing weight Italian style.

It's the secret I learned on the Isle of Elba and later experienced when I lived in Florence. Now it's becoming *your* secret.

R-E-S-P-E-C-T

Respect for food is nothing new. It's the original and most authentic attitude of human beings toward their source of nourishment. In ancient cultures when humans everywhere were more vulnerable to famine, food was considered sacred. People thanked the gods when it was plentiful, because they knew this gift could be revoked at any time, with dire consequences. Some people thanked the food itself for sacrificing its life and energy so that they could use it to survive.

Today, the majority of Italians conserve their appetites so that they can survive *and* thrive. They've learned that *enough* is as good as a feast. You don't see all-you-can-eat buffets in Italy. Italians prefer the feeling of being deeply satisfied to pigging out, and their discipline allows them to be relatively carefree eaters. There's nothing attractive or desirable about feeling stuffed and bloated. In other words, Italians know when to say *basta* ... enough. Overindulgence, oversaturation, whatever you want to call it, too much of a good thing really does kill the pleasure.

I've learned this concept myself, but recently I had the opportunity to watch it play out with a friend of mine. We were talking after dinner while he was eating a big bowl of ice cream. Suddenly he shoved it away with a look of disgust and said, "I'm not even enjoying it anymore." At the end of the meal, he didn't take time to gauge accurately whether he was still hungry. He just ordered the sundae. And rather than paying attention to whether he was enjoying what he was eating, he just mechanically (and mindlessly) kept downing mouthful after mouthful, beyond the point where the treat continued to taste good. What started out as being delicious suddenly sickened him because he ate too much.

People with a heart problem are said to have a bad ticker. I think people who have a troubled relationship with food often have a bad *picker.* Many of us have this problem. When your "picker" is broken, you have a problem with what you pick, both what you choose to eat and the amount you choose to eat.

Unstretching Exercise

Have you ever gone out to dinner and eaten too much, only to find the next day that you wanted more food than usual? It's occasionally happened to me. All I can think is that I've temporarily stretched my stomach. I don't know if that's what really happens from a physical standpoint, but Dr. Eldo E. Frezza, former director of the Bariatric Weight Loss Center at Texas Tech University Health Sciences Center, says in his own weight loss book that over a period of years your stomach actually grows if you eat too much. He says he's seen it with many of his obese patients.

When you eat too much food, your stomach becomes accustomed to larger quantities and won't be satisfied with normal portions. Your mind also becomes habituated to *abbondanza*. But when your appetite is raging out of control, it's hard to know what to do to get it back under control. There's only one thing you can do so that your body (and mind) learn to want less. You have to cut back on your consumption. But wait! This isn't a *bad* thing, it's a *good thing*. The least painful way I know to cut consumption is to eliminate all those "diet" foods that don't satisfy you anyway, and give yourself something better. Instead of miserably chowing down massive quantities of no-fat, no-sugar, no-good junk, indulge in reasonable portions of high-quality foods that you love so you don't feel deprived.

Be sure to eat slowly. And I do mean slowly. Savor each bite. I know this may be hard at first, but chew every mouthful forty times. Don't swallow a bite until you've done that. You not only obtain more nutrition from your food when you masticate properly, you *have* to take more time. This forces you to spend adequate time on a meal to allow for proper digestion and to allow yourself to feel full. What you'll find is, when you chew each mouthful forty times, you really may not want huge portions. You'll be satisfied halfway through your usual amount of food. This alone will revolutionize your eating habits.

Once you become accustomed to eating less, if you overindulge you'll know it. It's up to you to stop at that point. And you may not stop every time, at least not at first. But little by little, bit by bit, and bite by bite, you'll find yourself pushing away from the table when you feel full, not stuffed. And as you become accustomed to eating fresh, high-quality food and refine your palate, junk food will become less attractive. My experience is that it eventually becomes downright distasteful. You may indulge from time to time, maybe at some social gathering where there's nothing else on hand. But refinement of your taste buds will make you a more discerning eater. Think about some of the treats you enjoyed as a child and how they taste to you now. There's a world of difference between the flavor and quality of a kid-cravable, mass-produced ice cream bar filled with preservatives and artificial ingredients and a traditional gelato made with milk, sugar, and natural flavors.

I say go for the good stuff. Healthy food is very appealing when you're a healthy person. But it has to taste good. (That's why I'm writing about weight loss, Italian style rather than the grass diet.)

As a whole, Italians don't seem plagued by the problem of the broken picker. First, they're disciplined; and second, their meals include a naturally satisfying balance of carbohydrates, fats, and proteins that doesn't leave them vulnerable to cravings. And as for those Florentines that I was just talking about, in addition to not overeating, they also didn't snack between meals because it spoiled their appetites. Being connoisseurs of food, they delayed their gratification so they could fully appreciate the good food they ate … just three times a day.

Arrivederci to the American Mistake and Guilt, Too

A Sicilian friend of mine says no one ever ate snacks between meals when she was growing up in Palermo. "We never had snacks. Snacks didn't even exist." If anything, mothers gave children who found it hard to endure the long stretch between lunch at 1:00 PM and dinner at 8:00 PM nothing more than a piece of bread with a little bit of olive oil or sugar. When I first went to Italy, snack food didn't exist either. I remember wandering around one afternoon with a growl in my stomach and realizing that nothing was even open. The town was dead. The message was loud and clear. You weren't supposed to be wandering around eating in the middle of the day. You were supposed to be at home taking a nap.

Obviously, this isn't the case in America. For most of us, food is never more than a phone call or car ride away. And you'd better be prepared to apply your own brakes, since food outlets are ready to answer your "Feed me" call any hour of the day or night. Consequently, the delay of gratification made possible by eating better at regular mealtimes is one of the most important things you can learn from the Italians. You'll not only enjoy your food more when you do eat, you'll feel better about yourself, knowing that you are in control and can resist temptation. This one thing demystifies the eating process and makes eating and watching your weight a lot less frustrating. I brought this concept home to the States with me, and it's been the cornerstone of my own carefree weight maintenance ever since.

So forget about the idea of grazing and snacking. You're killing your pleasure and shooting yourself in the foot (also the hips, waist, thighs, and derriere). Snacking breeds more snacking and dulls your sense of taste. Give your digestion a rest once in a while. Get out of the habit and mindset that you need to eat all the time. It's what got you into trouble in the first place.

Do it the easy way. Eat only at mealtime. Eat foods that fill you up so that you don't snack on things that fill you out. Eat things that take a while to digest and learn to savor the feeling of longing as you work your way toward your next meal. Don't give in to twinges of hunger. Enjoy them for what they are—the spice that will make you appreciate your next meal all the more. Experiencing and identifying hunger and then holding off for something great at mealtime is one of the secrets to becoming and remaining slender. And the more you get used to it, the more you will be able to tolerate—and appreciate—it. If you allow yourself to go a little hungry instead of giving in to snacking, then you really do deserve a meal of foods you love, and you can guiltlessly enjoy it.

Evolution of a Naturally Healthy Italian

That same history of food scarcity that has made Italians respectful of food has also made the Italian diet a healthy one. This will assist your weight loss efforts also, and effortlessly so. The Italian diet is naturally low in animal fat because traditionally people could afford meat only on special occasions. Italians still eat very little of it compared to us. In fact, Italy's first cookbook, *Liber de Coquina*, written near the beginning of the fourteenth century, starts off with recipes for vegetables. Italians eat a diet that relies mainly on grains, fruits and vegetables, olive oil, fish, and legumes. That means their diet is high in fiber, which keeps a person full from meal to meal, inhibiting the desire to snack.

Scarcity also forced the Italians to be creative with what they had in order to make their humble eating experience as pleasurable as possible. Whatever people ate had to be tasty and hearty, and very satisfying. Learning to wring every ounce of flavor from whatever was available, cooks placed an emphasis on the quality of the ingredients. To this day the hallmark of Italian cuisine is its simplicity and freshness—things that make it such a pleasure to cook and eat.

As a general rule, ethnic restaurants aren't nearly as popular in Italy as they are in the States. It's not that Italians aren't adventurous from a culinary standpoint. It's just that they love their own cuisine above all others and never get tired of it. Who can blame them? You'll probably find the same thing. Enjoying the bounty of seasonal harvests and fresh-from-the-farm food choices, eating the Italian way is going to increase your dining pleasure as well as simplify your life. Italian-style food preparation is fairly simple, and once you've mastered the basic method you can do a million things with it. Just a few essential ingredients from the pantry are all you need to be able to whip up an Italian-style feast that's fast, easy, and pleasing to the palate.

The passion and care Italians put into their food is evident every step of the way, from the food growers to the sellers, the cooks, and the table where it's eaten. This is why you won't find pineapple pizzas in Italy. It's a weird combination that makes Italians gag because it shows no respect for the dish. There is even a national law that dictates what can be called an authentic Neapolitan pizza. (Neapolitan refers to anything that comes from Naples, considered the birthplace of Italian pizza.) Among other things, a pizza *Napoletana* must be round, not too thick, and no more than 13.8 inches across. It can only be made with extra virgin olive oil and tomatoes grown in the ash-rich soil around Mount Vesuvius.

Talk about attention to detail. It's this kind of fastidiousness that keeps Italians slim *and* well fed.

Not-So-Fabulous Fakes

Repeat after me: "*Poco, ma buono.* Just a little, but make it good." Adopting this as your mantra and putting it into practice will transform the way you view and experience food. A small amount of high-quality food eaten slowly is much more satisfying than a mountain of inferior junk. It's one reason why I'm not a fan of low-fat, no-fat, chemically-created "fake" versions of food that trick you into overeating. These things can actually cause you to gain weight. You see, foods that are low in fat are not necessarily low in calories. Sometimes it's just the opposite. Read the labels. When they take the fat out, they have to replace it with something else. That "something else" is often high-calorie, unhealthy processed sugar, corn syrup, or another sweetening agent.

I'm also skeptical of things with ingredients I can't pronounce or that sound more like they belong in a science experiment rather than your stomach. Regardless of how they taste in your mouth, these artificial foods aren't satisfying in the way real foods are. They make you want more, and you can end up eating more than you should because they're "diet foods." The result is a life of weight loss struggles.

Face it, if "fake" foods were really great substitutes—if a love affair with low-fat, no-fat versions of food really worked—wouldn't most Americans be getting slimmer? Yes … but American's *aren't* slimming down. We're getting heavier and heavier, and sicker and sicker. The empty calories of fake foods fill your stomach, but they do nothing to address your body's nutritional needs. Empty calories just leave you … empty.

And there's another problem. Processed foods do part of the work your stomach should be doing. Particularly if they're full of sugar, they break down and enter the bloodstream quickly. It's another reason we're so addicted to our food. Processed foods give you a lift, but it doesn't take long before you come crashing back to earth. Real, wholesome food on the other hand (like penne with broccoli, olive oil, garlic, tomatoes, and a shaving of cheese) takes longer to digest and makes you fuller longer.

I find whole grain pastas particularly satisfying at mealtimes. Some whole grain pastas have six or seven grams of fiber. That's staying power! When I eat a fortifying dish of pasta, I'm not hungry until the next meal. And on those rare occasions when I am hungry, I just eat a few pieces of leftover pasta. It's tasty, nonfattening, and quells the hunger immediately. Again, be sure to read the package label. Some products that claim to be whole grain include processed white flour. Look for packaging that says 100 percent whole grain.

Shifting to an Italian way of eating for me has meant ending my dysfunctional relationship with processed foods, fake foods, and anything fat free, sugar free, or low carb. In short, it's meant eliminating anything artificial from my diet. You want to know the result? Now that I eat only wholesome food on a regular basis, I can eat what I want. I'm satisfied eating three meals a day. I never count calories, fat grams, or carbs. I almost never snack, and I don't give one thought to overeating during the holidays. I've freed myself from that psychic torture. I *definitely* enjoy food, but I don't eat to excess. Like the Italians, I'm disciplined. I eat well at meals and therefore don't get hungry.

I Call It Wellpower, Not Willpower

Some people think I have incredible willpower. But it's not about willpower. It's just about eating well. Learn to eat the Italian way and you'll see. It eliminates the guesswork and you won't have to think so much. We tend to think of choices as a good thing, but having too many choices makes life stressful and can even contribute to depression. (For more on that, read *The Paradox of Choice: Why More is Less*, by Swarthmore College psychology professor Barry Schwartz.) Just make good eating a habit and your mindless eating will diminish.

It kills me when I see people torturing themselves over food all the time. It's so unnecessary! I remember how crazy-making it is to be in that kind of a relationship with food, and I'm thankful I'm no longer subject to it. When you approach food and weight like an Italian, you won't have to argue with yourself over whether or not you're going to have that cookie or whether every cup of coffee out with friends has to have a rich and calorie-laden pastry to go with it, or whether every trip to the store for groceries deserves some treat when you reach the cash register. You'll be able to forgo the popcorn, soft drink, and candy bars when you go to the movies. They don't have a place when you're eating a nice dinner afterwards—or have enjoyed a sumptuous lunch beforehand.

When you "go Italian" with your eating, you'll never starve yourself. As long as you eat your favorite wholesome foods in appropriate quantities at meals, you'll be in good shape, literally and figuratively. Satisfying yourself with *real food* will help you resist fakes, no matter how fabulous, and keep you from the Great American Diet Downfall—snacking.

The story of my friend Anne starts out as a tragedy of Shakespearean proportions, but keep reading. The ending is a happy one.

Anne's Story—Eating on Autopilot

Before Anne began implementing the concept of eating well at meals, she was in the habit of eating a lettuce salad for lunch in an attempt to try to keep her weight down. Maybe you've tried this, too, as a "sensible" approach to weight loss—to starve yourself when you thought that you could tolerate it. I'll bet you didn't have a lot of lasting success, did you? The idea usually backfired for Anne, too, because after fasting all day, she'd find herself making up for it at dinner. She was so hungry that she'd bolt down not one, but two bowls of low-carb chocolate ice cream. Where's the sense? Where's the nutrition? Where's the satisfaction? Gone out the window. Low carb doesn't mean very much when you sabotage your own efforts and down two big bowls of it.

Fast forward to Anne after she was bitten by the Italian diet bug. When she began to incorporate satisfying foods such as pasta into her meals, to her surprise, she no longer felt the need to snack. She wasn't even tempted to raid the freezer for ice cream, low carb or otherwise, because she didn't feel hungry. Slowly, Anne began to see the importance of nourishing her body instead of feeding it junk, regardless of whether she was trying to drop a few pounds or not.

Before she even realized it, Anne was paying more attention to the taste of her food. This may seem elementary, but it's surprising how many people wolf down their food almost without noticing and then wonder why they still feel hungry. Anne learned that to get the full effect out of it, her food needed to be chewed slowly and enjoyed. She became accustomed to the fact that it takes time for your stomach to let your brain know that it's had enough. It can't happen if you rush through eating and hardly even taste your food.

Starting to eat consciously represented a big shift for Anne. She said she noticed an important change one day when she caught herself shoveling hot zucchini into her mouth. She was so focused on just getting it down that she actually burned herself. *That* got her attention, and not in a good way. Later she caught herself standing by the kitchen sink gorging on a quart of blueberries. Remembering her reaction after the zucchini burn, Anne stopped gorging. She thoughtfully took one berry, chewed it slowly, and gave her full attention to its taste. She was surprised by how tart it was and wondered how and why she could have tried to eat a whole quart of them.

That was Anne's lightbulb moment. She realized how unconscious she'd been when it came to the food she put in her mouth. She'd been eating on automatic pilot, hardly even noticing what she was doing, and now she realized how often she'd overstepped the bounds of common sense. She said that as she stood at the sink with the quart of blueberries in front of her, she suddenly had the revelation, *I don't have to finish this.* Like many of us who grew up being admonished to "Clean your plate," Anne was astonished to realize that she was forty-three years old and was just beginning to learn that it was okay to say no to food.

Now Anne realizes she has a choice. She can eat unconsciously or pay attention to what she's doing. By paying attention she not only eats less, she's eating food that's better for her and enjoying it more. Anne has reached the magical place of moderation as she tunes in to her own intelligence rather than remaining a victim of impulse. This simple shift is giving her control over her food and weight issues.

Have you ever caught yourself eating unconsciously? Can you think of a time when you opened up a package of cookies, intending to have just one, and suddenly you found you'd eaten half the box? That's unconscious eating in action. If you'd noticed what you were doing and listened to how your stomach really felt, you would have stopped before you reached that point.

Italians do this. Their food monitor—their "picker"—isn't broken. So although they spend a lot of time thinking about food, talking about it, and eating with gusto, you rarely see morbidly obese people in Italy. Pasta, pizza, and gelato are prominent parts of the dietary landscape, but they're not eaten in excess. Italians eat small pizzas with crusts that are thinner than ours. They eat pasta in reasonable portions without rich sauces, and gelato is a treat rather than a requirement after a meal. (It's also made with milk, not cream.) They *don't* eat faux pizza made with tofu crust and dairy-free cheese, or any of the other things that are leaving Americans unsatisfied and, in some cases, obese.

Mangia, Good; *Mangione*, Bad (Glutton)

Food is the earliest sort of medicine. It is medicine, and taken the wrong way, in the wrong proportion, and at the wrong time, it can harm you. The Italians have a saying: *Ne ammazza piu la gola che la spada.* (Gluttony kills more than the sword.) A look at the number of health challenges that obesity causes confirm that notion in spades. A bad diet and a sedentary lifestyle are generally the root causes of weight gain. Until you come to grips with this and live your life mindful of what's true, a permanent change in your weight and health is next to impossible.

It's not for nothing that gluttony is considered one of the Seven Deadly Sins. The current obesity epidemic in the States is pulling down the average American lifespan. Obesity is the second leading cause of preventable death in the United States next to smoking, according to the Centers for Disease Control and Prevention. Former US Surgeon General Richard Carmona has said that if things continue as they are, the younger generation may turn out to be the unhealthiest in history and the first to live shorter lives than their parents.

And yet it's all so preventable.

Given what we know, why is it that Americans indulge in gluttony so frequently? My belief is that they eat not to nourish themselves, but to compensate for a lack of love, a lack of companionship, a lack of purpose in their lives, or because of a suppressed need for self-expression. Gluttons can't control themselves. They eat out of boredom and frustration, fear, stress, or a sense of inner emptiness. All of this "unhappiness eating" casts food in a role that it was never meant to have: a substitute for something else.

It broke my heart when I was in Italy recently to see a father buying his daughter a soda and potato chips on the train. Not so long ago that would have been unthinkable, but junk food is making headway even in Italy, and waistlines are expanding because of it. But it's still not seemly to be a *mangione* or glutton. Italians are very body conscious, and it's bad for the image to be plump. You know, the paparazzi are everywhere, and you can't have them catch you stuffing your face like a pig on the *Via Veneto*.

Still, gluttony can be sneaky. I was recently in a restaurant with an out-of-town colleague and ordered a chicken Caesar salad. My colleague, who said she was watching her weight, ordered a hamburger and french fries, then announced that we would share our meals. I wasn't interested in her hamburger and french fries. Fries are one of the worst things for you. Not only are they fattening, but fried foods aren't satisfying and make you experience hunger later. I'd seen her debating between the burger and fries and the Caesar salad, and rather than go for the healthy thing, she'd decided that she could have both by claiming some of mine. Her own plate of food wasn't enough. We've all been there, unable to decide between two things on the menu. But if you want other people's food, it's a sure sign that you need to start nourishing yourself better, or you'll be a glutton for life.

The Need for Greed

One of the embarrassing things about getting a handle on your food issues is facing and dealing with the greed factor. In the movie *Wall Street*, iconic figure Gordon Gekko says, "Greed is good." No, it's not. Greed comes from a place of fear that there's never going to be enough. There's no need to be greedy when it comes to food. We're not experiencing a famine. All you need to do to kill the need for greed is to promise yourself that you'll eat good food—wholesome food, like pasta and fruits and vegetables—at regular meals. You won't feel greedy, because you'll know when and where your next meal is coming from —a healthy, Italian-style kitchen!

Knowing when you're in this state of scarcity ("I didn't have breakfast") and understanding that it makes you feel hungry in a greedy way ("I'm starving and I don't have anything at home for dinner, so I'm going to stop for a double burger, fries, and a shake") takes awareness. Getting out of your greedy state simply requires patience. When you're overtaken by a deprivation/greed attack, pause and try to breathe your way through it. Try to understand the emotion behind it rather than diving for the food. There *is* enough. And you *will* get another chance to eat.

Eating the Italian way can help you overcome this. When you eat good food in proper proportions and shun junk food, you won't feel deprived.

The truth is, you can eat what you want. It just can't be all the time, and not all at once.

You Are the Boss of You

Italian society places great importance on looks and public deportment. And since obesity isn't as common or acceptable as it is in this country, family members can be hard on women if they gain too much weight. I don't agree with this kind of pressure, but it's probably true that living under the watchful eye of others can have a salutary effect.

If you don't have an Italian mother, father, or brother monitoring your trips to the refrigerator, you need to take 100 percent responsibility for your eating habits. That means being accountable to yourself for everything you put in your mouth. Otherwise you won't be able to trust yourself and reach the stage where you can become a carefree eater. It's when you can finally trust yourself that you can relax and feel in control of the situation. Until then, every eating opportunity poses a potential threat.

Some people have the mistaken idea that indulging in sweets is a way of loving themselves. I used that excuse, too, back when I was addicted to them. Sweets provide an artificial way of comforting yourself, but giving in to your cravings and treating every day as a food holiday is not loving yourself. It's the same as feeding junk to your pet. Fido may wag his tail with love every time you feed him the kind of human treat *you* would like, but you're shortening his life, which is not exactly loving.

I recently saw a woman at a drug store counter eating a gigantic banana split for lunch. My friends and I used to do the same thing sometimes as college students. But this was an older woman. Maybe she thought she was being nice to herself. Maybe her mom used to take her to the soda fountain when she was little. Maybe she thought it was no big deal to spend her lunch calories on the banana split. But it *is* a big deal. Poor nutrition and empty calories *are* bad for you. They break down the body and its defenses.

Shaking Sugar

Sugar is especially harmful in excess. If you don't believe it, read journalist Connie Bennett's book, *Sugar Shock!*, which details the debilitating physical and emotional effects a sugar habit had on her. The first winter I made my own decision to give up sugar, I never got sick once, and at the time I was teaching at a college. Do you know how many germs travel back and forth when you're teaching in a classroom, breathing the same air as thirty other people, and touching the papers of students who come to class with colds and flu? You have to have a strong immune system.

Not only is a banana-split's worth of sugar an assault on your system, those empty calories ruin your appetite for a nourishing dinner later. The above woman's ice cream dish was eight inches long and six inches high with its mountains of whipped cream. It was half the size of her head. She was eating alone, by the way. Was it a substitute for love?

Seeing this, I couldn't help remembering an ice cream parlor that was popular when I was a kid, where you could order an enormous "pig's trough." Only in America would this major detour from common sense be considered a good thing. I used to think it was quite a good thing, too. When I was little, I wished that I could live on sweets. I hated vegetables and would slip them under the table to the dog whenever possible. Visions of sugarplums danced in my head morning, noon, and night. Willy Wonka's chocolate factory would have suited me fine.

But that was then, and this is now. It's childish to think we always deserve a hot fudge sundae. You have to exercise your common sense even if there is none around you. Nobody needs food portions like that, least of all for dessert. Sad thing is, most people don't even know what a normal portion is anymore. You have to go to Italy to find out. Since you may not be going anytime soon, here's the Italian short course for portion control:

Nothing bigger than your fist.

Travel with a Chaperone

Italians don't go overboard. It's their discipline that allows them to enjoy food so much. Discipline is easy, *if* you have the right mindset. Don't view discipline as something distasteful or as a form of punishment. A lot of us shrink at the sound of it, because it sounds as if it will limit us. Actually, discipline is what sets you free. Free of worry so you can just be at ease and eat, no matter what the circumstances. Think of discipline as your strict but loving inner food chaperone. Drowsy chaperones may be hilarious on a Broadway stage, but yours needs to leave the bottle home and not fall asleep on the job.

So how is it that Italians maintain discipline when, at the same time, they're known for eating with such enthusiasm? They're brought up not to spoil their appetites. And they know the simple trick of putting a halt to their eating once they start to feel full. They don't continue until they're bloated. If you stop when you start feeling the warmth of satisfaction in your stomach and wait a little longer, that satisfaction will translate into a feeling of being full. This, also, is one of the best things you can train yourself to do. But you need to be eating slowly to know when you reach this point. If you rush through your food, you'll miss it and eat too much. Your chaperone needs to be on guard at all times.

Just Enough and Not Too Much

One of the benefits of eating slowly is that you truly find that you can be satisfied with a smaller amount of food. If you eat really slowly, chewing forty times, you'll be very satisfied with small pieces of whatever you eat, even modest slices of cheesecake and small servings of ice cream. Fine restaurants often give notoriously small desserts. It's the quality that counts.

So work on becoming a more refined person with a more refined palate, and opt for quality over quantity. Develop your subtle sense of taste. Learn to appreciate the flavors of real food rather than the artificial flavors and chemicals found in processed foods. It will make you healthier on many levels.

This, by the way, is the beauty of eating in courses. The time in between allows digestion to take place, and you won't want to eat so much.

If only Americans could grasp what the Italians know, that the time you spend on a meal and the quality of the food, not the amount you eat, increases your enjoyment. A meal stretched out over an hour or so with good company and conversation allows you to savor every morsel. Not everyone can take that long with their meals, but at least make yours an occasion instead of just ripping open a box of something or a bag or a can. If you have no one to eat with, you can still create enjoyable experiences for yourself by creating an inviting atmosphere and making good food.

You can also search out ways of making meals more communal and enjoyable by sharing them with others. Join a dinner club for a group meal once a week or once a month. Or organize one yourself.

Falling In Love with Food (and Out of Love with Snacking)

Are you ready to begin having a love affair with food? Before you do, you need to start loving yourself. By loving yourself, I mean caring enough about yourself to nourish your body with the best food and stop feeding it junk. Junk clogs up the system and interferes with your internal portion monitor.

You don't have to starve yourself. In fact, it would be unwise to do so since countless studies show that if you try to lose weight just by drastically reducing your food intake, your body will think you're starving. One result is that your body will hold on to its accumulated fat out of fear that there's no food to be had. Or you may lose weight, but when you normalize your eating habits, the weight may come back with a vengeance. Crash diets that promise to help you lose ten pounds in ten days ultimately crash and burn. Losing one or two pounds a week is more than adequate. Moderation is the key. Eat well, reduce your intake a little, and get more exercise, lots more exercise (or movement). Just make sure it's exercise that's pleasant for you.

Don't feel bad if you never understood the principles behind how to eat properly. You're not alone. Two-thirds of the country is with you. You probably didn't pick them up in your dysfunctional family or our fractured school system. (My sister once taught at a school where ketchup was considered suitable as the vegetable on the lunch menu.) But it's never too late. Another thing to consider about weight loss principles is the fact that everybody's different. I didn't understand the key to my own healthful eating and satisfaction until I went to Elba. While some people may seem to lose weight effectively on a program of diet and deprivation, I realized that for me the only way to maintain a trim figure was to eat and enjoy food to its fullest but in moderation, like the Italians. It was like learning to eat for the first time. I learned through practical experience that when I filled up on something satisfying like pasta, along with a nutritious fruit and a vegetable, I never felt the need to snack later.

Exquisite Agony

During a typical breakfast of coffee and *cornetti* at my hotel, the waiter would present diners with the menu for dinner so we could make our choices. The result was that we spent the entire day anticipating the pleasures of our evening meal. Regardless of what was going on, we knew we had something delicious to look forward to at the end of the day. Now, on Elba, most businesses close their shutters between 1:00 PM and 4:00 PM, and the only snack in sight can be found at a gelato stand. It's true I was sometimes tempted to have a gelato because dinner wasn't until 8:00 PM, but I certainly didn't want to eat much because I didn't want to ruin my appetite for the grand meal that was coming. And dinner *was* grand every night, a fun sit-down meal with friends, conversation, food and wine.

The hours between 4:00 PM and 8:00 PM were bittersweet. As the sun would start to set, I would feel the rumbling in my stomach that (in America) I would have satisfied with a snack. But in Italy, there was nothing available to assuage the rumbling. It became a pleasurable torture—exquisite agony—waiting for the dinner bell to chime. This was something I took back to Manhattan as a souvenir of my visit. I remembered and enjoyed the pleasure in feeling myself get hungry and making myself wait ... when I knew it was going to be worth it. This pleasurable "sweet longing" is the reason I urge you to cook for yourself and plan things that you're going to make so there's something wonderful to look forward to at the end of the day.

It makes all the difference.

The Rapture of Eating

Do you experience the rapture of eating, or do you rush through your food as if you're eating in a panic? Are you a glutton or an epicurean? To feel the real joy of eating requires a number of things:

- One, you must take your time.
- Two, you must slow yourself down.
- Three, you must have something good enough to feel rapturous about.
- Four, you must create an appealing and civilized atmosphere.

This is not about ripping open a bag of potato chips in front of the TV. May I give you some background and a "snapshot" of my experience? Here's what was rapturous about the eating on Elba, and what I tried to bring back with me.

It was an unbelievably sensuous experience waking up every morning to the sweet, intoxicating smell of those *cornetti* baking in the oven below my hotel room. It didn't matter how late I'd gone to bed the night before. It didn't matter that I was going through a divorce and there was no one in the bed beside me. I was having an ecstatic experience just lying there smelling the *cornetti* and fantasizing about what they were going to taste like when I got downstairs.

Breakfast was served on a garden terrace. There were flowers and birds singing in the background. This was also a time to meet with fellow students and talk before we went to class, so it wasn't like I was sitting there by myself, staring at my kitchen wall, which I would have been doing back home.

Cornetti on the Homefront

How did I recreate the Elba breakfast in Manhattan? I moved from staring at the wall in my kitchen to eating breakfast in the living room, a lovely space that was filled with morning sunlight. (I'm not sure why I hadn't thought of moving to the living room before. Sometimes it takes a trip to jar you out of your boring routine.) I also hung pictures of Italy around the house so that I could pretend I was on the island, even during a Manhattan winter. And I started using my good silverware and china. In other words, I was treating myself like a special guest, not a poor relation.

When I moved to California, I experimented with baking my own *cornetti*. The resulting disaster didn't dissuade me. I recreated the breakfast experience for myself at a local bakery/café that had tables under trees outside and some excellent French croissants that were close enough! (A numbers of Italians appeared to be eating there, too. I took it as a sign.) Croissants are high in calories, so I can't eat them all the time, or else I'll have the same problem I noticed right before setting off on my trip to Elba. But once in a while on weekends, a croissant at this bakery does the trick and helps keep me focused on the pleasures of weight loss, Italian style.

The point is that you need to make dining a pleasure somehow. It's not just about the food, so give yourself a pleasant surrounding, with pleasant company when possible, even if it's only on weekends.

The Divinity of Dinner

As a result of our smallish breakfast on Elba, we looked forward longingly to lunch and felt justified in eating it. On the days when I ate at the hotel, I remember walking up the beach, imagining the pleasure I was about to experience, dining *al fresco* on a delicious serving of pasta. Lunch was at 1:00 PM and dinner didn't start until 8:00 PM, so there was a long pause in between, during which, no matter what else we were doing, we all looked forward to a nice dinner together. It was a joy sitting on a swing in the garden and smelling the delicious smells of dinner wafting from the kitchen, then hearing the dinner bell and beginning to salivate like Pavlov's dog because I knew that something delicious was about to happen. The anticipation would grow as we seated ourselves at the table. I can still remember the crackling of breadstick wrappers being torn off as the waiters brought the wine. When they brought the food, they turned the plates just so, to best show off the dishes.

There'd be a first course, followed by a second course about twenty minutes later, plus vegetables or a salad. After another twenty minutes or so we were asked if we wanted dessert, which was either the specialty of that evening or a basket of fresh fruit, followed by coffee. It was gastronomic heaven, relaxation, and companionship all combined. And our hunger was quenched. Eating alone in Italy would be a travesty. It's a communal event. In fact, there's an Italian proverb that says, "He who eats alone, dies alone." Italians consider company at the table to be very important!

Dinner was a convivial time to break bread and discuss our day's adventures. It makes people happy and healthy to talk and eat food together at sundown. It's relaxing, and it brings a pleasant close to the end of the day.

And hunger really was the best spice.

Italian Dinner on American Shores

How did I bring dinner on Elba back to America? Well, after becoming accustomed to the delectable taste of fresh food, I knew I had to upgrade my eating habits, so I decided I needed to cook more for myself, using more care and better ingredients. I joined a food co-op where I received fresh produce. I also hung around some Italian restaurants and told the managers and chefs that I wanted to learn to cook. The managers didn't want me there, but the chefs were accommodating in the way you would expect of Italian chefs. They offered to give me private, individual lessons at home. I guess I could have killed two birds with one stone and gotten in the exercise element of the weight loss program while I was at it by having the chefs chase me around the kitchen, but I was really more interested in the food.

I *did* ask one Italian restaurant manager how he thought Italians stayed so trim and slim while eating what might be considered the best food between the sun and Jupiter. Without a moment's hesitation, he said, "We don't snack." That was it, pure and simple. His response verified what I'd seen in Italy. So I vowed to cut snacking out of my life, and I began to explore that feeling of longing for food instead of snacking, of nourishing myself well enough at lunch that I wouldn't be hungry in the afternoon, and planning things so good for dinner that I would look forward to it instead of ruining it by eating beforehand.

I've said before (and I'll say again) that snacking is the Great American Diet Downfall. Americans don't want to temper their appetites; they just want to enjoy eating. But what is consistently overlooked is the fact that the key to enjoying your meals, to losing weight and maintaining it once you reach your target, is controlling your appetite. Forgoing snacks means you can eat better at lunch or dinner. It's the healthy way to live. That coupled with choosing only the best there is to offer adds up to loving and enjoying food to its utmost.

You've Got to Have Friends

What else did I do to bring Italy to America? I missed the companionship when I came back to New York. So I threw some parties and had people over. It brought back that convivial atmosphere, and it was a great excuse to cook. When I moved to California, I took full advantage of the extraordinary produce available throughout the year. I did more cooking and went to Italy more often. I also became a member of Slow Food, an international movement dedicated to helping people reawaken the joy of eating.

You can join this, too. They have chapters all over the country, and events to go with them.

Good Enough to Eat —with Enthusiasm

I remember the Elba teachers, who lived together on the island, talking with great fondness about what they were going to make to eat one night—*spaghetti vongole!* It may be hard to imagine how a plate of noodles topped with shellfish could arouse such passion. But once you've enjoyed the delicate sauce of olive oil, garlic, parsley, white wine, and red pepper flakes, it's pretty unforgettable.

Then there was the night we went to a popular seaside restaurant. Three of the same teachers were talking with great gusto about what they were going to order, expressing such longing and anticipation over—not a hot fudge sundae, not chocolate cake, not a trough of ice cream—but *spaghetti vongole!* It was the same dish they'd made at home a few nights before, yet there they were salivating over the prospect of having it again at this restaurant. That's having a passion for food. They continued to salivate and talk about it as they waited for it to arrive at the table. And once it came, they oohed, and aahed, and sighed, and moaned until I thought of that scene in *When Harry Met Sally* and wanted to wave the waiter over and change my order, saying, "I want what they're having!"

Being Italian, I'm sure he would have understood and changed the order immediately.

So now, can you imagine one of the things I salivate over when I go to Italy (and dream about when I'm not there)? *Spaghetti vongole!* Of course it's good when I make it at home, too, but I'm not around a lot of fish eaters, so when I make it I have to eat it by myself, which isn't very *divertente,* or fun. Someday I'm going to invite a whole bunch of fish lovers over so we can sit around the pool and pretend we're in Italy. But you could do this sitting around a table with friends in winter in Chicago. The recipe is that good. (That's why I made sure to include it in the special bonus recipes you can download from my website at www.WeightLossItalianStyle.com/bonus.) The same thing is true of my Elba fisherman's recipe. They are, in fact, a little similar. Make sure you have some delicious, fresh and crusty bread on hand to sop up the sauce!

Savory vs. Sweet

Now I'm going to say something that may shock you. See, Tuscans have a savory palate—not as sweet as Americans'. It's a refinement that I enjoy. And after getting used to it and making pasta with high-quality extra virgin olive oil a staple in my diet, I've lost my obsession for sweets. Believe it or not, I would really rather eat pasta, which I do several times a week. And because I do, I rarely find myself craving anything. The only time I get enthusiastic about sweets now is when my mother, who is a great cook, makes something fantastic, or if I'm at a birthday celebration or a party. It's nice to eat them then, because it's a rarity and part of the celebration. But it would never occur to me to buy ice cream or cookies or such at the store unless I'm having company.

To get to the point where you prefer real food to ice cream, cakes, cookies, and pastries—or any kind of junk food—you have to first experience, then fall in love with the taste of good food itself. And to enjoy these delicate tastes, you must get in the habit of buying the freshest food you can.

Hard, hothouse tomatoes don't hold a candle to those ripened on the vine. And bagged bread can't compete with fresh bread from the bakery. You know what's good and what's not. And what's not should never go into your mouth.

Portions and Eating in Courses

The rule of thumb for slim, naturally healthy Italians is *never eat anything bigger than your fist.* (I grew up with the expression, "Never eat anything bigger than your head!") This means small amounts of lean meat or fish, not a rack of ribs or a slab of beef. It means one or two pieces of bread, not the whole loaf. It's a great way to gauge your intake without the nuisance of counting calories. It's so simple. Counting calories is a pain and is not a normal way of eating, anyway. A healthy person should be able to simply look at food and gauge how much they can eat. You can enjoy vegetables in abundance, and a very small dessert, if any, completes the meal.

Once you've got a handle on portion control, you'll find that eating in courses gives you time to digest your food and allows you to feel full. In our country there's not enough of a pause between courses to digest your food because, well, we don't dine in courses when we eat at home. And when we do eat at a restaurant, often they whisk away the plate and bring on the next thing as soon as you're done. You need to have a little time between the soup and salad and the main course, and especially before dessert. If you wait and digest your food, you probably won't even need dessert. Scientifically speaking, it takes about twenty minutes for your stomach to tell your brain, "I've had enough."

Rushing through meals makes you fat. Eat in a leisurely fashion when you can. The time you spend on a meal increases your enjoyment of it. Eat slowly, and savor every morsel. Eating fast is like unsatisfying sex. It's perfunctory and goal oriented. It's a little like skipping to the end of a good book. The pleasure's in the reading and the anticipation, not just in knowing how it ends.

Size and Season Matter

Size matters! Don't use gigantic dinner plates. Studies show that you eat less food on a smaller plate and drink less liquid when it's in a tall, skinny glass.

Be sure to read labels. If the ingredients sound like a science experiment rather than something you'd want to put in your body, don't. (I was once told how to get rid of cellulite: eliminate all processed foods, commercial baked goods, fried foods, and sugar from my diet and add fish oil. I tried it and it seemed to work.)

Eat with the seasons, taking advantage of what Mother Nature provides, which is what's best for you at any given time of year and when it also tastes best. Strawberries in winter may be nice for a treat, but it's really more satisfying to eat them when they come out in summer. They taste better. It is their time.

You can also turn everything into a positive. Instead of, "Oh, no, I can't eat cheesecake, it's so fattening," here's the new rule: "Great, I love cheesecake. I'm going to have *a bite*!" Eat that one bite slowly, and enjoy it.

Make these habits permanent. That's the only way you can become a carefree eater, because life is always going to find ways of tripping you up with parties, vacations, and birthdays, etc. Your habitual good eating habits will carry you through times of temptation and stress.

Your Action Plan—Steps You Can Take *Now*

I don't like homework, but I do like results. If you bone up on the strategies below, when you go to Italy (or anywhere else for that matter) and you're confronted with the most common Italian date question, "Want to go for a pizza?" you'll be able to respond with gusto and absolutely no guilt, "*Certo!*" (Certainly!)

So let me encourage you to:

Live like an Italian:

- Exercise discipline.
- Don't eat anything bigger than your fist.
- Don't avoid good food. Engage with it openly, in moderation.
- Buy quality ingredients.
- Eat delicious food presented nicely, in small portions. Less is more.
- Savor your food.
- Eat slowly, in courses if possible.
- Explore your local farmers markets.
- Join the Slow Food movement. (They may have a chapter in your area.)

Keep a Food Journal

This can be *very* instructive. Use your little pocket notebook from Chapter 2 and write down everything you eat on a daily basis until you break the habit of eating between meals. Wear a pencil around your neck if you have to. Then you won't "forget" that extra cookie or that taste off someone else's plate. Or licking the bowl, or raiding the refrigerator, or taking samples at the grocery store. *It all counts*, and writing it all down so that you can see exactly what you're eating in black and white (or whatever color pen you use) is illuminating.

Read through your notes at the end of the day. Your goal is to eat so well at meals that you stop snacking.

Clean Out Your Pantry

Go to your pantry right now and toss out the processed food and junk food. That would include all the things full of preservatives and additives or any items with things on the label you can't pronounce. You want to be eating food in its purest form.

If you can't stand to throw these things away, package them up and donate them to your favorite charity or food kitchen. Walk or ride your bike. If you must take the car, park far enough away that you get some exercise carrying your load of goods.

Teach Yourself To Buy, Cook, and Eat Fresh Ingredients Only

Take pleasure in seeking out farmers markets or wandering through the fresh food section of your grocery store. It's almost always on the periphery, right when you walk in. The deeper you go into the store, the more unhealthy the food gets. So stay on the outer edges, except for the olive oil and pasta aisle.

You get a better workout walking along the sidelines, anyway. And you'll find most of the things you need there, including fresh produce, fish, eggs, bread, and wine.

Create a Beautiful Space for Eating

Aesthetics are important. A beautiful environment relaxes you and prepares you for a leisurely, digestion-friendly gastronomic treat. It doesn't have to be elaborate. What can you add to make your meal a dining experience rather than just a refueling opportunity? How about some flowers in a vase? A candle to soften the mood? A pretty tablecloth and napkin? A little night music?

Practice the Art of Affirmations

The power of the mind can be redirected with affirmations. Affirmations are positive phrases that you repeat over and over to plant the seeds of success in your mind. As an Italian-style eater, your food mantras should be:

- "I eat three times a day, and I eat well at meals."
- "I can have what I want, just not all the time, and not all at once."
- "Hunger is the best spice!"

Take a Moment to Look Before You Leap into That Food

Really look at it before you dig in. There's pleasure in doing this. Notice the presentation. Is it attractive? Does the food look good? Does it smell good? Does inhaling stir your gastric juices? Give every item its due share of attention. Notice the different textures and colors. Do they please your senses?

This would be a good time to thank the universe for this life-sustaining meal.

Savor the Flavor

When you eat, you should take a small bite and really taste your food. Close your eyes and savor the flavors. Let your taste buds do their thing. Give them a chance to please you. Chew that mouthful forty times. Swallow and take a breath before you take your next bite. Remember, anything in excess causes problems, so you need to pay attention to the tipping point and stop before you get there. If you become sensitive to the subtle energies of your body, you can actually feel the effects of various foods. Tune into your inner awareness. It will tell you what feels nourishing and how much to eat.

Leave the Table Hungry

Sit back and stop eating as soon as you feel the warmth of satisfaction in your stomach. You don't need to eat until you're full. Leave a little room.

Make Fruit Your Friend

Perfection is an ideal, not a reality. When the inevitable moment hits and you feel you must have something for dessert, try a piece of fruit instead of something sugary. And before you swallow it all in one great gulp, consider eating it the European way, peeling and slicing it with a knife. It's meditative to sit at the table and peel your fruit. It gives you time to contemplate what you're going to eat and to appreciate it. (And if the fruit's not organic, it takes away some pesticides along with the skin.) The first time I was introduced to this, I thought it seemed like a lot of trouble. But once I got used to it, I liked it, because it prolongs the pleasure of the meal.

Chapter 4:

On the Move

Nevertheless, it moves.
—Galileo

One of the first things foreigners notice when they visit Italy is the sense of movement and life happening all around them. People get up early and move throughout the day. They walk after dinner, and the piazzas buzz with activity after sundown. Italians know how to move! Vitality is in their genes. (Not just their jeans.) Next to their eating habits, the number one reason why Italians are slimmer than Americans is because of the amount of exercise they get in their everyday lives.

If you want to lose weight and keep it off, you need to bring that sense of vitality into your own life and move like they do.

Now, you could drop the weight by starving yourself, taking drugs, sweating to the point of dehydration, or destroying lean muscle mass, but these methods are drastic and dangerous. The best way is to modify your eating habits and get more life-enhancing exercise. And I don't mean just until you lose the weight. I'm talking about a permanent lifestyle change. Not some flash-in-the-pan weight loss for the holidays or your summer vacation. We want results as lasting and eternal as the city of Rome.

Diet junkies who only think in terms of losing pounds miss the point, often believing that once they reach their weight loss goals they can relax and go back to their sloppy habits. They can, but the weight will come back. That's why only 6 to 10 percent of people who lose weight are able to keep it off. Most dieters don't understand the secret to weight loss longevity. It's this: instead of focusing on losing weight, put your focus on becoming healthy. That means making exercise an integral part of your life—something you can't live without. The easiest way to do that is to fall in love with it.

Car Culture

The sad reality is that for the most part our convenient American way of life revolves around cars and does not provide enough natural exercise opportunities to keep a person healthy, let alone fit and toned. Two-thirds of Americans are overweight at the moment. The World Health Organization estimates that by the year 2015 the figure will be more like 80 percent of the adult population. How can you avoid becoming one of these statistics or pull yourself out of the pool if you're already there? Not by going on some awful diet, which I'm sure you've already tried. Instead, do what the Italians do. Start moving your body.

Think of what you're doing as moving rather than just exercising, because it ought to move you physically *and* emotionally. Movement needn't be a chore. It can be a pleasure—a passion, even. It ought to be fun! If you were Italian, moving would be easy. You couldn't escape it. Did you know that Italian women get more exercise than American women just by virtue of living an Italian life? They burn off calories by walking and going up and down stairs. They get weight-bearing exercise just by shopping and lugging home their groceries.

Your sedentary lifestyle may seem normal to you until you go somewhere else and see how other people have to move just to get along in life. That's what happened to me when I went to Italy and dropped weight without even thinking about it. It was so easy to stay in shape there that I realized I wanted to continue living that way for the rest of my life, even if I wasn't in Italy. I knew that weight loss, Italian style would mean that I wouldn't have to worry about love handles or worse—what one teacher on the Isle of Elba graphically referred to as "sandwiches beneath the behind"—the things that had sent me reeling in the first place.

Bodies in Motion

There's a way to avoid those, or get rid of them if you already have them.

Remember, Italians only care about three things—beauty, food, and love (and, okay, sex)—so they know about this. Falling in love with movement *all'Italiana* is the way to make staying in shape seem effortless. There's beauty in moving your body. Think of it as the cultivation of grace. When I used to work in the restaurant business, we always talked about saving steps. But in weight loss, Italian style, the more steps the better!

Some people just abhor the idea of having to exercise. They cringe when they realize they've got to get up off the couch and move. Believe me, I've been there. When you're not accustomed to exercising, the thought of it can seem pretty distasteful. But having discovered the joy of moving, I know that when a person dislikes the idea of it, they're simply looking at movement the wrong way. Movement increases your health. Your body can't function properly unless it moves. Movement also increases your pleasure quotient.

Most importantly, trying to lose weight without moving is an uphill battle. Lack of movement is the reason why many dieters fail.

Bodies were not meant to sit around all day. My yoga teacher says that if you don't move, the fluid surrounding your joints dries out, causing you to become stiff. Who wants to dry out? The last thing we need is to become less juicy. So, the sedentary life has to go.

While I don't like to focus on calories because people become obsessed with them, it's useful to realize that you need a deficit of 3,500 in order to lose one pound. To achieve this, you could eat a lot less, but if you starve yourself without exercising, your muscles start to atrophy and your metabolic rate may decrease, making it even more difficult to lose weight.

You could eat what you normally eat and increase your activity level *a lot*, but that's pretty difficult for most people. What works best is a combination of both. Increased movement helps you lose weight more efficiently, and it makes you feel less sluggish, more alert, and more fabulously energized. It puts a spring in your step and a sparkle in your eye that others can't fail to notice.

I know that starting an exercise program isn't easy. Your body and your mind want to resist, and that initial resistance is the most difficult part. Once you push through it, the process of moving regularly becomes easier, if not pleasurable. The trick is not allowing yourself to put it off, because if you procrastinate, you'll end up waiting forever. Days become weeks, and weeks become months, then years. Want to know the right time to start exercising? The right time is *now*.

View movement as a life enhancement tool that will tone your body while melting off the pounds. View it as your Italian-style beauty booster. Regular exercise is one of the two main things that will allow you to eat the relatively carefree Italian way.

American Women Transformed

In America, many young women experience what's called the "Freshman Fifteen," a fifteen-pound weight gain during the first year of college. Living on their own, too much food, and too little exercise become the order of the day. American co-eds who head off to Italy, however, have another experience entirely. A language teacher in Florence told me that many, if not most, American students (male and female) begin shedding weight within their first few weeks of living in Italy. A teacher at a fashion institute related that it wasn't unusual to see some go from a size sixteen to a size ten or sometimes even an eight during the course of their year abroad.

American girls drop weight because they don't have cars and have to walk everywhere, including up and down hills and stairs for the first time in their lives. They have to carry groceries and lug their laundry to laundromats. And they have to do it constantly. Many complain about it in the beginning. But do you think they're complaining when they get their brand new, sexy figures or when men say, "*Ciao, Bella,*" and really mean it?

Life in the Kristi Lane

Take, for example, Kristi, who lost weight while studying in Florence, despite her notorious sweet tooth.

"My family is well aware of my passion for food, and somewhere in the back of their trained-to-hate-carbs American minds, I think they expected me to return to the States with a bit more of 'me' than I left with," she said.

But even with all the pasta and bread she ate, she didn't gain weight.

"I'm sure I could have returned dramatically thinner if I'd tried, but I didn't try. I enjoyed myself to the fullest. What amazes me is that I did not gain weight after consistently indulging as I did."

Kristi would start a typical day by descending five flights of stairs to have a cappuccino down the street at her favorite café. Then she'd stop by a market for a couple pieces of fruit. She had to climb stairs to get to her class, and afterward she'd walk a few blocks to her favorite pastry shop for a blackberry pastry. Then it was off to another class and up another few flights of stairs. After working in a photography darkroom, she and her friends would head over to a supermarket for a bag of oranges and some salmon and cheese and crackers, or they'd go to their favorite sandwich place for pesto with mozzarella, turkey, and tomato sandwiches on warm foccacia, or some other Italian delight.

In the afternoon Kristi had another class a fifteen-minute walk away. In class she'd snack on some nuts, and afterward she'd walk half an hour to the other side of town where she worked. Later she'd walk half an hour back to the other side of town, where she'd meet her roommates for a dinner—usually *pesto gnocchi* or *ribollita*, a traditional Tuscan soup, preceded by bread dipped in olive oil. Afterward they'd buy gelato and eat it while strolling around town.

"Some days I'd have two cappuccinos. Some days I'd have two pastries. But some days I wore a pedometer and found that I'd walked seven miles without even realizing it."

Kristi said that after examining her habits, she believed that the reason she lost weight and felt healthier in Italy was because of "consistent, sometimes rigorous exercise that didn't *feel* like exercise. It was just part of a day of living." Kristi could enjoy pastries and gelato frequently "because I was burning the calories from them simply by moving throughout the day."

Kathryn's Story

Another American woman, Kathryn, lived in an apartment at the top of a four-story building in Florence.

"There was an elevator, but it was locked, so we had to use the stairs. All day long it was up and down, up and down. At first it was like, 'Oh, my God, I'm not gonna make it!'"

There were stairs to climb everywhere else in the city also, since most Florentine buildings are hundreds of years old and don't have elevators. Kathryn *did* get used to it and said that when she returned home only one month later, her family was surprised by how much thinner and healthier she looked.

"In Italy, you're constantly on the move."

And, she found, the Italians eat differently.

"Here in America, we eat when we're happy and when we're sad. We eat to celebrate and to reward ourselves. When we're depressed we go to the pantry and eat chocolate chips. And here we have twenty-four-hour access to food. We're impulsive. You can wake up at 3:00 AM wanting chocolate chip cookies, get in the car, and go. They don't have little mini marts open every day in Italy. There, some stores aren't even open on Sunday. And on weekdays they close at 1:00 PM and don't open until 4:00 PM."

Students who go to Italy live in apartments with small refrigerators. They do their shopping on foot or by bicycle and don't have as much access to junk food or fast food as in the States or the cupboard space in which to keep it. The time they used to spend sitting in front of the television is spent walking to school, walking to do their shopping, walking to do their laundry, walking to museums, or walking to meet friends for dinner, drinks, or gelato. Rather than watching the boob tube, they're outdoors engaging in life.

As Kathryn learned, in Italy she was forced to move constantly in her everyday life because she didn't have a car, and she burned off far more calories than she ate. My Italian friend Rudy learned a similar lesson.

Rudy, who now lives in America, spent a month in Italy once and came back eight pounds lighter, despite the delicious food. He was staying with a friend who lived next door to his girlfriend, and they went to her house for all their meals. He said it was "up the stairs for breakfast at Bice's, then down afterward. For lunch we went up and down again, and again for dinner, up and down. You know how many calories you burn going up and down? And if you forget to get something at the store, you have to go back down again, and then back up."

The stairs weren't just good at forcing people to think twice about going shopping; they were good for the glutes. And all that good movement made all that good eating possible. It's why Italians are so healthy. Rudy said of his former countrymen, "Their metabolism is excellent. They drink a lot of wine and do a lot of walking. And their food is pure. No preservatives."

Be a Food Hunter and Gatherer

With some effort, you can create this part of the Italian experience in the States. Will it be torture? No. Once you make moving Italian style part of your life, it makes your existence much nicer. As I sit down to write this, I've just returned from an hour's shopping excursion to my local Saturday farmers market. It was invigorating to get out of the house early in the morning. And it uplifted me to walk through my neighborhood at that time of the day, looking at people's gardens and admiring their trees and flowers. It got my blood flowing, I was breathing fresh air instead of sitting indoors, and I knew I was doing something good for myself.

It was pleasant wandering through the food stalls, interacting with the vendors and sorting through their produce for my weekly needs. Open-air shopping brings you in contact with your neighbors and your community. I take special joy in perusing the colorful displays and imagining what I'm going to make with all the fresh fruits and vegetables.

Sure, it takes longer to walk to the farmers market than to drive to my local supermarket. But it's more gratifying. And walking and carrying groceries takes care of my exercise requirements for the day. I can eat what I want for breakfast or lunch, because I've burned my calories. I feel good because I've taken care of myself and at the same time supported local growers. I feel a connection with the land, and seeing the fresh produce stimulates my desire to cook delicious and nutritious meals.

In Italy, people are constantly on the move like this, whether it's going to work or doing their daily shopping. You don't have to make an effort to go somewhere and physically exert yourself at a gym—unless you want to. People shop, run errands, and visit friends on foot. Even with public transportation, they still have to walk and climb stairs. (Women in Italy have one other advantage, although some would say a disadvantage depending on how you look at it, and that is that they have to walk pretty fast to keep ahead of Italian men.)

I experienced the stair-climbing phenomenon myself. When I lived in Florence, I climbed eighty-eight steps to and from my apartment several times a day to go shopping, to attend language lessons, and meet friends for gelatos and cappuccinos. Just lugging my suitcase up the stairs to the apartment the first time worked muscles in my legs I didn't know I had. My calves and glutes ached every time I went up those stairs. But I not only got used to it, *I loved it*. I welcomed that climb, because it meant I could eat what I wanted, and it put me in great shape so that I didn't have to worry about those "sandwiches beneath the behind." The only sandwiches I had in Florence were the great panini I ate at the city's delightful cafes. Scaling those eighty-eight steps so many times a day was what made all those cappuccinos, panini, pastries, and gelatos possible. I loved those steps!

I was never that fond of math, but I thought of movement and eating in the following parallel equations:

Lots of movement = I could eat what I wanted

or

Sit around on my duff = develop "sandwiches beneath the behind"

So again, the question is how can you apply the Italy experience to your own life? How can you replicate that amount of movement in the States so that you can enjoy relatively carefree eating and still lose weight? I was wondering the same thing when I returned to New York after my first experience studying on the Isle of Elba. Among other things, I didn't want to give up that feeling of burning off my meals so efficiently. But I knew that whatever I came up with would have to be simple; otherwise, I wouldn't stick to it.

Let's Pretend

My method? It couldn't get much simpler. I just pretended that I was in Italy and decided that I had to move like an Italian, which meant to move and move and move.

Pretend and you're halfway there!

Fortunately, New York is a walking city, so I walked from one side of Manhattan to the other, across Central Park, from the West Side to the East Side to go to doctors' appointments, and down Broadway to do my shopping. I walked across the park to the Metropolitan Museum of Art. (The Museum itself is so big you can put in miles of walking just looking at the different displays.) I walked down Park Avenue to attend functions at the Italian Cultural Institute. Occasionally I'd even walk back home from Midtown when I had to see my lawyer—forty blocks. I put in so many miles that if there'd been a "frequent walker" program, I might have earned enough points to take me back to Italy.

I cooked more at home, but on the occasions when I did go out to eat, I ate well and sometimes walked back instead of using a taxi. By walking like an Italian, I did my part for the environment by cutting down on pollution, and I put in more than enough exercise to allow me to occasionally indulge in fabulous meals in New York's Little Italy (where you can find Lombardi, which officially became America's first pizzeria in 1905).

Other entertainment money went toward dance classes. Instead of only going to movies and watching others move on a screen, I learned to move my own body. This was an electrifying experience, because in New York City you can take lessons from world-class teachers. Dancing opened up a whole new universe. It provided me with a passionate new form of exercise and a mental rest from the legal hell of ending my marriage. It also afforded me an intriguing new venue for socializing. Dancing boosted my confidence, gave me poise, and kept me in contact with the opposite sex in a nonthreatening way. It was balm for the soul while I was going through a divorce.

City Mouse, Country Mouse

That was my life in the city. But what do you do if you live in "car country"? I'm glad you asked that question, because when the divorce was finalized, I moved back to California and found myself in precisely that situation. I was living in the suburbs and for the first time in over twenty years had the use of a car. My goodness, was that convenient! I no longer had to lug around groceries. I didn't have to schlep in the rain. The only movement I had to do on any given day was to push my shopping cart up and down the aisles of the grocery store, and even then they had little motorized vehicles if I got really lazy. I thought I was in heaven, but hell was just around the corner.

Before I knew it, I was living a life of lethargy. My blood seemed to stagnate, and it was hard to work up the motivation to move. I was developing calluses on my behind and probably on my mind, too. It was at that point I realized that I was going to have to get some exercise, or I was going to once again be a resident of Sandwiches-Beneath-the-Behind Land.

What could I do? The easiest and most obvious: I went back to pretending that I was in Italy, which wasn't that hard, considering the climate in California is much more Italian than New York's. I got back into walking, even in car culture.

Walking is really one of the best types of exercise and one of the easiest. The reasons are endless:

- You don't need any special equipment.
- You can do it just about anywhere, anytime.
- It gets you out in the fresh air.
- You get to experience nature and hear birds singing.
- You don't have to stick to anyone else's schedule.
- It works your muscles, gets your blood pumping, and makes your bones strong.

The other beauty of walking as your chosen exercise is that you can always fit some type of walking into your daily routine, whether it's a morning walk, an after-dinner walk, or a simple walk around the block. My eighty-three-year-old father regularly walks to the store to do light shopping. About once a week, he and my mother and I walk to a café near my house for coffee and a pastry. Sometimes we walk in the late afternoon or after dinner. They go walking in a park on weekends. If people in their eighties can do this, certainly the rest of us can manage it.

Walking is the exercise of choice for people of all ages everywhere in the world.

Kathleen's Story

My friend Kathleen used to walk five miles on a treadmill at the gym until another friend mentioned that he needed to exercise, too. They decided to start walking together after work. It gave them time to talk about their day. Within ten or fifteen minutes of starting their exercise they'd be feeling better, and by the end of their walk they'd be rid of all the stress from work. They settled into a routine of walking for an hour or so and covering three-and-a-half to four miles Monday through Friday ... and five miles every Sunday, unless it was pouring down rain.

"It's much more fun looking at all the neighborhoods than walking on a treadmill," Kathleen said. "Especially at Christmas, it's so pretty with all the lights."

Once a week they walk to their favorite restaurant, where they share great food and a bottle of wine. "One night we had too much and ended up singing all the way home!"

Kathleen says that walking this way helps her to keep her weight steady. "And I feel better. Psychologically, it's very good, too. It wasn't much fun doing the treadmill. Now if we don't walk, it really bugs us. And you process what you eat better. You aren't as hungry when you get regular exercise. But you can actually eat more."

Walking regularly allows you to experience the joy of a healthy, hearty appetite. The last time I was in Rome, we grabbed dinner at a sprawling Italian-style cafeteria above the train station when we returned from a trip one evening. I was amazed to see the enormous spreads of food in front of the Italian travelers. Almost all of them had a pasta first course, a second course of meat or fish, a salad, a vegetable, bread, a beverage, and water. Even under such casual circumstances, they still dine like kings. And the reason they can eat that much is because they *need* to. They walk—a lot.

I wanted to know more about the benefits of simple walking. So do scientists.

When You Go Walking, So Do the Pounds

Scientists have long wondered why the Masai of Kenya and Tanzania have such a low incidence of cardiovascular disease, considering their high consumption of animal fat. At first it was believed that they were genetically protected against it. But a recent study suggests their secret is the vast amount of walking they undertake as a seminomadic people. The Masai, known for their erect posture and elegant gait, walk long distances on a regular basis. They also suffer few back or joint problems, which may be related to their active, walking lifestyle.

Don't worry. You don't have to leave home and become a nomad in search of a healthy figure. The National Weight Control Registry, which keeps track of thousands of people who have shed thirty pounds or more and kept it off over a year, has found that most successful people start out by walking on a regular basis.

There are many ways of approaching walking as a form of exercise. Again, don't worry. You can start small, especially if you're not in the habit of exercising or if you are very overweight. In fact, it's important to consult with a health professional before embarking on any kind of diet, weight loss, or exercise program to find out what's appropriate for you and your unique situation.

No one likes a bully, and that includes your mind and body. Both will respond better if you start slowly and work your way up to a good routine. Don't push yourself too hard in the beginning. Make a commitment you know you can keep. The best one *I* know? It's a commitment to simply being more physically active each and every day. You could start with twenty to thirty minutes of walking a day. Maybe take a walk after breakfast or dinner.

If that seems like too much, just walk as often as possible to get you into the swing of moving like an Italian. Start moving like an Italian and you'll start becoming like an Italian—in other words, more active, attractive, and able to melt off your meals.

Once you start moving, you'll find lots of opportunities to keep moving everywhere. Make moving during the day as automatic as brushing your teeth. Walk to the store. Walk to a coffee shop on weekends to meet friends. Walk on your lunch break. Whatever you do, just keep moving. If Americans would simply walk on a regular basis just for the pleasure of it, or if they carried their grocery bags—filled with luxurious ricotta cheese, buttery mozzarella, fresh fruits and vegetables, and pasta, pasta, pasta—they'd be in much better shape. Who knows? With the ever-fluctuating cost of gas, we may start to see more and more Americans leaving their cars at home and using their feet for commuting.

As someone living Italian style, in the spirit of the Renaissance, you need to be creative. You can walk to an art museum. You can walk to the market on weekends. You can walk on your lunch break. In the rain you can walk with an umbrella or walk at the mall.

Let walking get you outside. It boosts immunity, lowers blood pressure, and releases those pleasure-giving endorphins that make you even more vibrant and alluring. It lifts your spirit. And when you notice the admiring glances of strangers who can't help but notice *you,* your spirits will soar!

You can adopt the Italian ritual of *la passagiata* if you have a location that lends itself to it. *La passagiata* is the ever-popular evening stroll. It's a golden time when you can grab a gelato or a glass of wine, watch other people, and be watched. In Italy it provides the opportunity to show off your latest outfit, new pair of glove-soft leather shoes, or a new love interest. Think John Travolta in *Saturday Night Fever* when he struts in Brooklyn.

Scale Down Your Weigh-Ins

Whatever you do, make your walking enjoyable. Stay focused on the *pleasure* of walking rather than any weight loss that may occur. In fact, I have a suggestion for you. It's radical, and you may even find it a bit shocking. I encourage you to put your bathroom scale in the back of your bedroom closet and forget it even exists.

You don't need a number of pounds and ounces to tell you whether your body is in good shape. You don't need a scale at all. It's the self-judgment machine, and the judgments it hands out can be pointlessly devastating. Scale watchers are obsessed with day-to-day weight loss. That's not what's important to most Italians, and it shouldn't be important to you.

You're losing weight and developing a healthy body for a lifetime. You're in this for the long haul. Instead of letting daily weight fluctuations send you into a panic, monitor your weight by how your clothes fit. Monitor your health by how you feel. Do you have more energy? Do you no longer lose your breath walking up a short flight of stairs?

People who are addicted to the scale judge themselves harshly depending on whether they lose or gain a pound or two, when this is not very important in the overall picture. It's *normal* for your weight to fluctuate a little. Besides, muscle is more dense than fat, and as you develop lean body mass, you may actually stay the same weight or even gain a little, even as you begin to look thinner and your clothes become looser.

Weight is not the issue. It's how you look and feel that matters. If you looked like _____ (fill in the blank with your favorite curvalicious beauty), would you care how much you weighed? In fact, do you know what various celebrities weigh? Does it matter? They just look great. *That's* what matters.

If you depend on what the scale says, a temporary weight glitch has the power to discourage you and even destroy your progress. So stick with the program. Some well-known programs insist on weekly weigh-ins. But when you're doing things Italian style, weighing yourself once a month is quite sufficient. *Va bene.*

Step It Up

America on the Move Foundation, a nonprofit group that urges Americans to develop healthier habits, says that you can stabilize your weight or reverse the American trend of gaining one or two pounds a year simply by adding two thousand steps to your day and cutting one hundred calories. One hundred calories is about a pat of butter or a few bites less at meals, according to some estimates. That's easy.

And the two thousand steps? If you'd like to achieve them, here's what you can do. Buy a pedometer and strap it on when you get up in the morning. Wear it for a few days to figure out the average number of steps you take each day, then add two thousand steps. It's not that hard. Just walk around the block once or twice or commit to longer walks for your pooch. Walk all the way across parking lots instead of parking right in front of the store. Better yet, walk to the store.

You think you don't have time to walk? Take your cell phone and use your phone time to walk. (I've seen people chatting on the phone at the gym while they do their circuit. Yes, it's obnoxious, but that's another subject.)

Other experts say that ten thousand to twelve thousand steps a day—about five miles—is the magic range for losing or controlling weight. (The old number was ten thousand. Now some are saying it's more like twelve thousand.) I can wrack those up just walking to my farmers market and back on weekends to stock up on fresh basil, garlic, and other local goodies for my Italian-style kitchen. A pedometer is great for keeping track of these high figures. Start wearing it in the morning, and if at the end of the day you haven't put in your requisite number of steps, pull on your boots, throw back your shoulders, and start walkin'.

Turn Off the A/C

As you may have gathered, life in Italy is anything but convenient, and that's a good thing if you want to lose weight. American culture is a monument to the easy way, but there's a flipside to that coin. Italians don't enjoy all the everyday conveniences we do, but most of them don't have the weight problem we face, either. And there's a relationship between the two.

After I moved to California, research took me back to Italy yet again, where I lived in Florence for a while with a cooking teacher near the top of a very old palazzo built during the Renaissance. Once a week my landlady was down on her hands and knees scrubbing the hard wood floors of her sprawling apartment. I was expected to keep my part of the place clean the same way. Now, the heat can be extreme in Florence. It leaves no doubt in your mind where Dante, a Florentine, got his idea of the Inferno, and this was one of the hottest summers on record. I didn't relish being down on my knees scrubbing floors in one hundred-plus degree weather with 90 percent humidity.

There was no air-conditioning, not even a fan in that grueling heat. Like a lot of Florentines, La Signora didn't seem to believe in them. So, we sweated it out. You've seen those people who try to lose weight sitting in a steam bath? That was us. But you know something? Mopping that floor by hand in that weather caused me to lose weight. Easy, no. Effective, yes. And it's good for the skin and body to sweat once in a while. It flushes toxins, for one thing. And all that activity, plus sweating buckets, earned me my late-afternoon or late-evening gelatos at my favorite gelato shop—the one with the picture of the Mona Lisa hanging behind the counter and the view of the Arno River.

And while I don't believe that air conditioning causes obesity, I did come across a study conducted in 2006 that suggested that widespread use of air conditioning and heating can contribute to fat build up by requiring the body to use less of its own energy to warm up or keep cool.

The lack of air-conditioning at La Signora's also caused me to spend my evenings outdoors, walking around and taking advantage of Florence's substantial summertime nightlife, since it was too hot in the building to go to bed before midnight. The streets of Florence were alive with people laughing and enjoying themselves. On the same kind of night in my old New York or California neighborhoods, everyone would have been in couch-potato mode.

I'm not advocating a return to the Stone Age or being victimized by extremes in temperature. I'm just pointing out that relying on conveniences can backfire. If you're not doing your own housework, washing your car, or doing your own gardening or laundry, just what *are* you doing to give your body its natural, normal, *appreciated* workout? What kind of routine exercise are you getting to make up for it? For many of us, the answer is, "Not much."

Well, you need to do *something*. You need to move. And then you need to keep moving.

I work at home, in front of a computer, and had been getting down on myself for my habit of becoming distracted. (I have ants in my pants and move from room to room a lot.) Thanks to the Italians, I realized this is not a bad thing. It all counts as physical activity, including my walks to the kitchen to make a cup of coffee—with whole milk, by the way, if I'm making a cappuccino.

Even cooking and everyday housework require you to move. My eighty-year-old mother has always attributed housework, cooking, and gardening to keeping her limber, and I guess she's right. I think she may be Italian at heart!

You may think this sounds silly, but apparently it matters. And it all falls under the idea of living as naturally as possible, just like the Italians. (When in Rome do as the Romans. When at home, do as in Rome!)

I'm Not a Freak

Just for the record, I'm not an exercise freak. I don't particularly like grunting and sweating at a gym. I have a membership, but I haven't used it lately, and when I do, I'm pretty dainty with the weights. But I've trained myself to have a healthy mindset where exercise is concerned. Both your mind and body need it. I hate that sluggish feeling of malaise I get when I miss my walks, and it just makes it harder to get out the door the next time. That's why it's important to be consistent.

It's how I look at exercise that has gone from American to Italian. I no longer complain that I *have* to exercise. I'm thrilled that I *get* to exercise. It's a privilege to move your body. Just ask anyone who is confined to a bed or wheelchair or who has lost the use of their limbs. I know from my own painful experience what it's like to be confined to a wheelchair and not be able to go outside, and it's like being in prison. We take it for granted that we can walk, but not everyone can. Walking is a gift. We're lucky that we can move our bodies, especially out in nature, and we should take advantage of it. And when those feel-good endorphins start to kick in and you become accustomed to them surging through you, you miss them when they're on vacation. They are the reason why some people become addicted to exercise. If you've got to be addicted to something, it might as well be that instead of food.

So, move out of the disease of lethargy and into the new world of moving throughout the day like a sexy Italian. Fitness, poise, and fluidity are second nature to *la bella figura*.

Okay, so you can walk and climb stairs. But why leave it at that? I take a half-hour walk every day after dinner in the summer and before dinner in the winter. In nice weather I ride my bike to do my shopping in the morning. Stretching is important, so I do yoga. Yoga also calms you down and destresses you so you're less likely to eat. I also like martial arts, but I haven't actually done any within recent memory.

I have that gym membership, which I haven't used in several months. But I want to. If you don't have the discipline or really don't have the time to go to a gym, throw on some music and get out your weights at home and lift. I have some weights lying around. Those I *do* use. I am in my best shape when I go to the gym three days a week and lift weights. But I haven't had time to do that in the last three months, so I've been using my weights at home during work breaks. It's easy, it's fun, and the main thing is I do it. When my work gets less intense, I'll go back to the gym. It's important to do some weightlifting for your bones and muscles and so you don't develop that saggy-baggy look as you drop the pounds.

Here's the part I really want to drive home. There's a hard way to lose weight, and there's an easy way. The hard way is every way you've tried and failed at before. And we don't like those. They're not the Italian way. The easy way is, on top of walking, find and fall in love with some fun activity you can do a couple times a week. Develop a passion that burns calories and fat. Or develop several so you don't get bored. Do as Joseph Campbell said and "follow your bliss."

What makes you happy? What thrills you? What do you think is fun? What did you like to do as a kid? Roller skating? Ice skating? Playing a sport? I'm as lazy as the next person, but I make movement a game, a fun and passionate game that I always get to win. My favorite additional exercise is dance, because it feels more like ecstasy than exercise. Any kind of dance is great, but I love Latin dance best. It's high energy, it's fun, and you get to wear great clothes!

If that doesn't turn you on, there's also ballroom and swing. There's line dancing.

Just fall in love with some sort of exercise. It will change your life. You'll look better. You'll feel better. Plus, it gets you out of the house so you have something to do on Friday night.

If You Don't *Have* Time—*Make* It

Now a word about time. I know time is becoming a scarce commodity in our society, as precious as diamonds, but there's still some of it going around. Maybe more than you're willing to admit to. That's why I need to ask you: do you have time to exercise?

As you think about your answer, think also about one of Florence's most famous characters, Pinocchio. Is your nose getting longer? Are you really being honest about how much time you have to exercise? Because the truth is that when it comes to exercise, you have to *make* the time.

It might seem like a challenge to fit exercise into your daily routine, but if you lived in Italy you would. If you had to shop on foot in order to eat, as many Italians do, you'd find a way because you wouldn't have a choice. And you might actually enjoy it, because it would stir things up a little and bring you into contact with the outside world.

When can you fit in that fun sort of exercise? What do you do in the evenings? How about the weekend? If I offered you a million dollars, I'm sure you could find the time. You'd do it for the money, but will you do it for yourself? This is where push comes to shove. It's a test of self-love. Because on some level not loving yourself properly got you here in the first place.

There are people who have time to go to movies, watch TV, get their hair and nails done, go to restaurants and socialize with friends, but they just can't find the time to exercise. And that's okay—if you don't want to lose weight. If you do, however, then there's something wrong with this picture. Life is a series of choices. In every moment you have the choice to become the person you want to be or to remain as you are.

Becoming healthy has to be more important than having your nails done. It has to take precedence over television and going to the movies. Physical activity has to be at the top of your "Things to Do" list. You have it in you to become what you want if you make it your priority. To do that you have to start identifying with the powerful part of you that can *initiate change* rather than being best friends with the lazy, stuck part.

Don't be surprised when the movement of your body creates movement in other areas of your life. Decide to do active things on dates instead of just sitting around over a meal or drinks. Can't find a date? Could it be because you're not exercising? It's not your weight or size that's keeping you from dating; it's isolation. All the activities I've been talking about bring you into contact with other people.

One last tip: People tend to be enthusiastic in the beginning, then at some point become disillusioned or frustrated or impatient with an activity—especially when they hit a plateau. And then they give up. You can avoid this pitfall by engaging in an activity you love and by setting realistic goals. Slow and steady wins the race. It's not about doing anything fast. It's just about being persistent and doing it.

Don't be hard on yourself like a drill sergeant. Be gentle, loving, and firm, but flexible and forgiving, like an Italian grandmother. If you mess up and fall out of your routine, just pick yourself up and get back on the bicycle.

Your Action Plan—Steps You Can Take *Now*

A Day in My Life

This is a very loose example of how I structure my days and make sure I get enough exercise on a typical weekday or weekend day. Sometimes I switch things around, but you'll get the general picture.

- Wake up
- Eat breakfast
- Get some exercise
  - Take a walk
  - Go for a bike ride
- Work and keep moving
  - Play around with free weights during breaks
  - Stand up while talking on the phone
  - Take frequent breaks to walk to the kitchen for water
- Eat lunch
- Get some exercise
  - Walk around the block
  - Work with free weights
  - Touch my toes
- Work
- Make dinner
- Get some exercise
  - Take a walk
  - Go to a museum
  - Dance class
  - Yoga
  - Make love (whenever possible!)

A Day in Your Life (Today)

Use the area below to write down *how you spend a typical day* from the time you get up until the time you go to sleep. No cheating!

A Day in Your Life (Tomorrow)

On *this* page write down how you are going to move throughout the day like a sexy Italian. Include formal things like adding in a dance class, yoga, or a martial arts class, but also walking time and ways that you are going to include informal movement into your work day, such as walking around while you're talking on your *telefonino* (cell phone) instead of sitting. Be sure to include a list of new, fun types of exercises you can explore a couple of times a week.

Chapter 5:

Pasta Is a Girl's Best Friend

Everything you see, I owe to spaghetti.
—Sophia Loren

In her delightful cookbook, *Sophia Loren's Recipes & Memories*, Ms. Loren tells an amusing anecdote about how she often startled interviewers by telling them she maintained her figure by eating pasta. She admits it was only a slight exaggeration because she does, indeed, love pasta and eats it nearly every day.

Need I say more? Pasta is one of my favorite foods, too. When you eat it, you don't get hungry between meals. You won't find yourself rooting around in the cupboards like a hungry bear. There's no need to raid the refrigerator, as it short-circuits the desire to snack.

It's *pasta, e basta!* (Translation: pasta, and no more!)

Pasta Never Made Anyone Fat All By Itself

Put down pasta, and some Italians put up their dukes. I can still remember La Signora, my landlady in Florence, pounding the kitchen table and shouting in indignation, "Pasta never made anybody fat!"

As a cooking teacher and an Italian, she took it personally that Americans were singling out pasta as a "bad" food choice for people who wanted to lose weight.

"It isn't the pasta that makes people fat," she insisted. "It's what they put on it and how much they eat. It is not the fault of the pasta!"

Looking at Italians, many of whom eat pasta every day, or even twice a day, I have to agree. You couldn't prove it by me, either. I ate it all the time in Italy, and I never gained weight. I lost it. That's why I made it a staple in my diet when I returned home, despite the high-protein/"carbs will kill you" craze.

The no-carb craze hasn't hit Italy yet, and probably never will. Italians love pasta. It's entrenched in their national identity. Pasta is not only tasty, it provides a healthy blend of carbs and protein, vitamins, and fiber. It fills a person up but it doesn't fill them out.

In Italy, if you don't have pasta noon and night, you feel as if you haven't eaten. (All right, now I'm the one who's exaggerating—just a little. In northern Italy, they eat risotto also. But everyone still loves pasta.) It's usually the "first plate" in an Italian meal, followed by a course of lean protein. And you can also have it as a main course if you add some vegetables and eat it with a salad.

Don't take my word about the wonders of pasta. Consider the facts. The average Italian eats more than sixty pounds of pasta a year, according to an Associated Press report. Many won't go a day without eating pasta. Some compare it to poetry.

And Americans? We eat one-fifth that amount, according to Fortune magazine. What do we consume instead? More than 30 pounds of cheese, for one thing, according to the International Dairy Foods Association, and 24.5 pounds of candy, according to the US Census Bureau. In fact, *Sugar Shock!* author Connie Bennett suggests that Americans may eat up to 170 pounds of sugar a year, or nearly a cup a day. And we think pasta makes people fat? Good grief, Charlie Brown! No wonder the spaghetti-loving, risotto-eating, fettuccine-feeding Italians are slimmer than we are!

Pasta is the key to helping me maintain my weight. I eat it all the time. Many people believe that pasta will kill your diet. But I'll even go out on a limb and say that pasta can be your best weight loss friend and weapon. It's low in calories—yes, you heard that right—yet filling, plus it's nutritious and easy to make. And it comes in so many varieties and is so versatile you could cook it every day for a year and never eat the same thing twice.

But, you might ask, aren't carbs bad for people who want to lose weight?

Carbs, Necessary and Not Evil

Carbs are not evil. They were not sent from the Underworld. Your body needs them. The US Government recommends that 45–65 percent of our daily caloric intake should be made up of carbohydrates. Why should you love carbs? Because carbs such as pasta are a great source of energy. This is one of the reasons why Olympic swimmer Michael Phelps used pasta to help catapult himself toward multiple world records and a chestful of gold medals. High-quality durum wheat semolina and whole grain pastas have staying power, and their low glycemic indices mean they give you a slow, steady supply of fuel while allowing your blood sugar to stay constant so you won't get hungry between meals.

The kinds of carbs you *don't* want to be eating are the very things that most people grab: refined carbs with a high glycemic index. Foods such as cookies, cakes, and all those other goodies break down quickly during digestion, causing blood sugar levels to spike and then plummet, which results in feelings of hunger. High glycemic foods are believed to induce cravings. Eaten at the end of one meal, they can cause you to want to eat even more a short time later.

Quality pasta isn't in this category. Unlike overcooked pasta, pasta cooked *al dente*—the way Italians like it—has a low glycemic index. And the effect of eating it is, in my opinion, nothing short of miraculous.

When I incorporated pasta into my diet on a regular basis, my cravings ceased. You, too, will feel fuller longer on pasta than on many other types of foods, especially if you eat whole grain varieties. When your body is satisfied because it's been given the nutrition it needs without any of the junk it doesn't, you won't be tempted to snack. This is why I think of pasta as dream food for dieters, salvation for the slim conscious, and a blessed relief for the taste buds. Pasta is what I define as a "perfect" food: low in calories and fat, but dense and chewy and satisfying. Pasta is something you can sink your teeth into to get that deep feeling of contentment that mealtimes should provide.

So, why does pasta get such a bum rap in weight loss circles? It's based on a misconception. When Americans think of pasta, many think of heaping plates of noodles swimming in rich sauce or covered with meatballs. Present that picture to an Italian and she'll say, "What is that?" When Americans think about pasta and Italian food in general, they're usually thinking about the *Americanized* version of Italian food, like those canned spaghettis that sound Italian but are strictly American. Italians would *never* eat any kind of pasta out of a can.

An American-style pasta diet can indeed make you fat. It helped me put on a tummy. As I write this, I'm remembering of one of my favorite "Italian" restaurants in Manhattan, a big, boisterous place where the pasta and meat dishes came on such enormous platters—with massive desserts to follow—that I used to feel like I was at an Italian wedding. Such portions are the epitome of the Italian spirit of *abbondonza* and generosity, and something that would be enjoyed for a special occasion. Overloaded plates of rich lasagna with heavily buttered garlic bread and sweet ricotta cheesecake is not what Italians eat every day. Not if they want to stay thin.

So how did the American version of Italian cuisine evolve? And how did wonderful, nutritious pasta come to be thought of as the Diet Devil's favorite tool? To understand that, we need to look at history, most specifically, the history of pasta.

A Taste of Pasta History

First of all, there are two basic types of pasta—hard and soft. The one you are probably most familiar with is the hard type. It comes in a box or cellophane wrapping and can be stored in your cupboard without refrigeration. Hard pasta, from which we get the majority of all those delectable spaghettis, linguines, rigatonis, pennes, and the like, is made of durum wheat, which comes from the south of Italy.

On a recent trip I was privileged to meet Giancarlo Gonizzi, curator of the Gastronomic Library of Academia Barilla in Parma, which maintains more than eight thousand volumes on Italian cooking. He told me that little documentation exists on the history of pasta. "No one knows for sure when or where it came from," he said. "There is no real history or proof, just little bits and pieces of information."

I was intrigued and wanted to know more. I was already aware that the Romans made dough from flour and water, which they flattened into sheets called *lagana*. These were sometimes cut into strips and cooked. From Mr. Gonizzi I also learned about a picture on a tomb from the time of the Etruscans (about 700 BC) that shows a person using what some believe to be pasta utensils. It's one of many wonderful pasta history stories floating around. But it turns out that the charming story you may have heard about Marco Polo introducing pasta to Italy by bringing it back from China has no basis in truth. How can I be so sure? It turns out that during the years of his absence, a man in Genoa wrote a will leaving a case of macaroni to his heirs.

"We know that the Arabs had the habit of using pasta because it was easy to carry in the desert and easy to dry out in the sun," Mr. Gonizzi told me. He said it's generally believed that dried pasta, which was good for carrying long distances, came to Italy with the Arabs through Sicily, although no one knows when it arrived on the scene or where.

If you'd like to know even more about the history of my favorite, and perhaps *your* favorite food, I've posted an article on my website: www.WeightLossItalianStyle.com/articles.

Italian Pasta

Sicily is the first place where we have evidence of durum wheat pasta—the kind of hard wheat that Italians eat so much of and that is the most common in America. Soft pasta made with egg is characteristic of the north of Italy.

If you think all pastas are created equal, you probably haven't been exploring them to any great extent. The range of quality is quite surprising. And the shapes are amazing: spaghetti, angel hair, penne, wagon wheels, orecchiette, shells, and even novelty pasta in shapes for kids … and some just for us grown-ups.

Don't Settle for the Same Old, Same Old

For me, and I hope you, too, one of the joys of eating pasta involves experimenting with different brands, which broadens your eating enjoyment and guarantees great satisfaction at meals. My favorites are the real Italian pastas, imported from Italy. Italians are insanely passionate about the quality of what they eat and insist on only the best ingredients. That's why their food generally tastes better than ours. If you haven't tried them yet, you'll find Italy's artisan brands of pasta to be flavorful, with a more enjoyable texture than many American counterparts, although there are definitely American whole grain pastas that have great flavor, too.

Flavor? Yes, flavor. You didn't realize that pasta has a flavor? There's a good reason for that. Since American-style pasta—especially the kind in "quick meal" packages—isn't known for its flavor, cooks tend to drown it in a lot of fattening sauce.

It's true that most pasta is made from just two ingredients, flour and water … but not just any kind of flour. Italians insist that their pasta be made of semolina milled from hard durum wheat (the word for hard in Italian is *duro*), which is harder than regular wheat. Pastas cut with soft wheat such as farina tend to become mushy and fall apart when cooked. They have no texture and can't be cooked al dente, or "to the tooth"—that delightful, slightly firm, yet chewy consistency that makes pasta, well, toothsome—the way Italians like it.

Italians eat pasta, not pablum!

So the quality of the flour is one factor. Another difference between a premium dry pasta and an inferior, boring product lies in the skillful blending of durum wheats (an Italian specialty) and the drying process. (No. Not all pasta is fresh in Italy. That just wouldn't be practical, and it's a different type of dish.) The great durum wheat pastas undergo a slow and careful drying process at low temperatures, which preserves their flavor as well as their nutritional value. The area around Naples, where pasta used to be sold on the streets and eaten by hand, has an excellent climate for drying pasta and is still home to numerous producers. The better manufacturers don't rush this process.

But wait … there's more. Premium Italian pasta producers make much of the source of their water and credit it with providing flavor to their product. This is true also in Abruzzo, a relatively remote and unspoiled region across the Apennines from Rome. Even in June, when I traveled to that part of Italy, the mountains were stunningly snowcapped. This region is home to producers such as De Cecco, Rustichella d'Abruzzo, and Delverde, which all attribute the flavor and quality of their pastas to the delicious taste of their pure water from mountains or springs.

Finally, unlike cheaper brands, high-quality pasta is "extruded" or pushed through perforated bronze molds or plates known as "dies," which create the different shapes. Cutting pasta with bronze dies gives these quality pastas their characteristic coarse texture. It's this rough surface that grabs onto the sauce. The sauce naturally adheres to the pasta instead of ending up at the bottom of your bowl, so you don't need as much of it. Try that with glossy white noodles! From now on, look for gold-hued pasta with a dullish surface that will cling to the sauce.

For all these reasons, premium imported pasta *is* more expensive than most domestic brands. Some artisan brands are quite a bit more expensive. But it's worth investigating the higher-priced pastas, because the pleasure you extract from your experience will be that much greater.

Why *Al Dente?*

Most Americans have explored pasta beyond the bland, canned versions that were so popular decades ago. But even though our tastes have broadened, we continue to make several major blunders when it comes to preparing pasta. These mistakes are costly because they rob us of the exquisite pleasure that is good pasta.

To the Italian mind, our cardinal sin is overcooking. The pasta must be cooked al dente, which means it still retains some substance. In fact, it should still be slightly firm in the center.

Why is al dente important when you're trying to lose weight Italian style? Because you want something you can sink your teeth into, something with texture that gives you the full sensation and satisfaction of eating. You want to chew your food, not gum it to death like a toothless person hunched over their bowl of gruel. Overcooked pasta doesn't provide any pleasure to the senses. It's not particularly fun to eat.

There's another reason why you should cook your pasta al dente. Italians believe that pasta cooked al dente is healthier for the body and the digestive system than squishy, overcooked mush that sits heavy in the abdomen and makes you feel sluggish. When it's overcooked, pasta has absorbed its maximum of cooking liquid. Al dente pasta, on the other hand, can still absorb more water during the digestion process and therefore digests more easily. It also has a lower glycemic index than overcooked pasta, so it will make less of an impact on your blood sugar levels.

Perfecting Your Pasta

Cooking pasta is easy as one-two-three. First, pasta should be cooked in plenty of water. Americans often don't use enough. Figure at least one quart for every quarter pound of pasta, or four quarts for a pound, if you're going to measure. All I can say is use a big pot and lots of water! You want the water to return to a boil quickly after you add the pasta; otherwise it takes forever to cook. Copious amounts of water also give the pasta room to move and to cook evenly and prevent the pieces from sticking together. Lastly, you need a lot of water because the pasta is going to double in size by absorbing it.

Now for the salt. I use sea salt, and I'm always careful to wait to add it *after* the water starts boiling. If you add it at the beginning, the abrasive action of the salt may pit your cookware before it dissolves in the water. Cooks differ on how much salt to use. I like what Sophia Loren says. Use a "large pinch." Too little salt leaves the pasta bland, but too much will overpower it. (In general, Italians will tell you that you should enjoy salt and everything in moderation ... except, I guess, for *amore!*) I usually just pour salt into the palm of my hand and see what looks right. You'll learn to judge the right amount as you experiment like an Italian cook, who goes by instinct.

The Taste Test

Now comes the tricky part: knowing when you've achieved al dente. Now please! Don't go throwing ribbons of fettuccine against the wall to test for doneness! As fun as it sounds, Italians don't do it that way. Not that the Italians aren't fun loving. They just know that if your spaghetti sticks to the wall, you're in trouble. It's overdone.

While pasta manufacturers usually have cooking directions that give approximate timings, you can't rely on them completely because there are so many variables. You really need to taste a piece. That doesn't sound too bad! What I usually do is add the pasta to the salted water, give it a stir, and set the timer. And then I always check it before the timer goes off. It should be just a little tougher than you like to eat it, because it will continue cooking as it drains.

Portion Control!

The Italians have given us "strike one" for the way we cook our pasta. The second cardinal sin of Americans, and the one that gives pasta its reputation as a dieter's nightmare, is our habit of eating too much pasta at one sitting.

One of the reasons why Italians have the luxury of eating pasta every day, or even twice a day, without gaining weight is because their portions are modest. In Italy, two ounces of dry pasta is considered a standard portion if it's served before a fish or meat course. If the pasta is going to serve as your main dish, figure three ounces—four if you're really hungry. (You may find two ounces a bit skimpy, unless you're eating lots and lots of vegetables, which isn't a bad idea.)

I usually just eyeball it or cook the whole box and save whatever I don't eat. And I don't care what anyone says, unadorned pasta cooks up great—and fast—as a leftover. Just dump it in boiling water for thirty seconds, drain, and eat it with your favorite sauce.

If you cannot trust yourself yet, then boil up only as much pasta as you are going to eat at each meal.

Three Strikes and You're Overweight!

The third cardinal sin of the American-style pasta eater is making sauce, not pasta, the star of the show. Don't drown your high-quality pasta. It spoils the experience of tasting and enjoying all the subtle flavors of good pasta. Plus, in most cases, it's the sauce that adds the calories. Believe it or not, a couple tablespoons of a thick sauce is sufficient for a bowl of pasta. The sauce is meant to enhance the pasta, not overwhelm it. Think of it as dressing your pasta in a light wrapper, not a heavy winter overcoat.

It's not the sauce that makes the pasta. You can definitely dress a good pasta in nothing more than high-quality olive oil, and it tastes delicious. I do this all the time. All you really need to make a meal are some vegetables. One of my most memorable experiences of pasta was when we were staying in Rome and had returned from an exhausting day of sightseeing outside the city. My boyfriend, John, had picked up a panino on the way home. (A panino, you remember, is the wonderful Italian version of a sandwich.) I hadn't eaten anything myself, thinking I'd save my appetite for a nice dinner later.

By the time we got back to our apartment, however, I was too tired and too hungry to make a proper meal. Or so I thought. In my pantry, I found a box of unopened pasta. Premium Italian-style pasta. I boiled it up and dressed it with the only thing on the shelf, a little bottle of Peppoli olive oil, an exquisite artisan quality brand made from hand-picked olives in Tuscany.

You can't imagine how good it tasted! The sounds of pleasure I was making made John curious. He asked what I was eating, and I gave him a taste. One was not enough. He ended up eating an entire bowlful. This wasn't the first time I'd cooked pasta for John. But it *was* the first time I had used this particular quality of pasta and olive oil, and he still remembers it as the best he's ever tasted.

One of my favorite quick meals to this day is to boil pasta, throw in some vegetables during the last couple of minutes, drain, and drizzle it with extra virgin olive oil and a sprinkling of grated parmigiano-reggiano cheese. (I got this from an Italian, so it's really okay.) Add a little cooked meat or seafood and you've got your protein, starch, and veggies for a meal that cooks up in the same amount of time as it takes to cook the pasta.

Getting Fresh

No discussion of the wonders of pasta would be complete without a celebration of fresh pasta. Made of soft wheat flour and eggs, fresh pasta is identified with northern Italian cooking. It's fun and easy to make it yourself if you have plenty of time and enjoy cleaning flour off your floors and counters. Fortunately, fresh pasta is readily available in many grocery stores nowadays. It has a tender consistency and cooks in half the time as the dried variety. Fresh pastas, like ravioli or tortellini, come stuffed with meats or cheeses and are richer than the dried kind, but they're convenient, delicious, and nice for a change. Since they're richer, adjust your portions accordingly. They're good with the lightest of sauces. A little butter or olive oil and a touch of seasoning will do just fine.

To meet modern health needs, many pasta makers now offer organic, multigrain, gluten-free, flaxseed, and even rice-based varieties of pastas. Farro, a grain popular in the ancient world and said to have fed the Roman legions, is enjoying an encore in Italian cooking. While most Italians eat regular pasta, I like to experiment with the other varieties, including whole wheat. They can be an even healthier choice since they have twice the fiber. For this reason, they're excellent when you're watching your weight, because the extra fiber slows down the digestive process and keeps you fuller longer.

Many of these new varieties are delicious in their own right, but they tend to have stronger tastes and heartier consistencies than Italy's standby and may require a stronger sauce, or "fashion statement." I like them fine just with extra virgin olive oil, cooked broccoli florets, and a sprinkling of cheese.

It seems that every time I go into my local specialty store I find a new variety of pasta to try. Selezione Monograno Valentino Felicetti, a high-quality artisan brand, produces organic durum wheat pastas as well as other delicious varieties, including farro, kamut, egg pasta from free-range hens, and spelt (a grain so popular with the Romans that they offered it to the gods). As you expand your horizons, just be careful not to overcook these whole grain varieties even a little, because if you do they'll become soggy.

I've already mentioned that I'm not a fan of snacking because it ruins your appetite for the main event. But if you absolutely must snack on something, a few pieces of plain, or better yet, whole grain, leftover pasta from the refrigerator work wonders. They'll curb your appetite and hold you over until your next meal without the downside of processed snacks.

How to Eat Spaghetti

You've bought premium Italian spaghetti. You've cooked it al dente the way the Italians do. Now comes the good part: eating it. Like everything the Italians do, eating spaghetti is a passion, an art that I learned the hard way after messing up a fine white hotel tablecloth with flecks of red sauce.

To eat spaghetti like an Italian, you need to focus on what you're doing—not a bad thing, because it makes you slow down and eat with attention. Twirl two or three strands on the tines of your fork—slowly, so you don't flick the sauce all over the place. You can do it nonchalantly against the edge of your spaghetti bowl. This is why a wide, flat bowl works better than a plate, although once you get the hang of it, a plate will pose no problem.

Do not twirl your spaghetti against your spoon. A European friend told me it's the way the prisoners do it.

In my humble opinion, but I think the Italians would back me up here, the best way to eat spaghetti is lip-to-lip, a la *Lady and the Tramp*. Who can forget that romantic restaurant scene beneath the stars, when the love-struck pups unknowingly suck the same strand of spaghetti from opposite ends and wind up kissing?

Just don't wear a white shirt.

Your Action Plan—Steps You Can Take *Now*

- **Try eating pasta at least once a day** in appropriate portions, and see if it doesn't curb your desire to snack. Use two ounces if it's part of a meal, and limit yourself to three if it's the main course. Four only if you're really, really hungry.
- **Experiment with delicious, high-quality Italian artisan brands** and extra virgin olive oil.
- **Let the pasta speak for itself.** Use only a couple tablespoons of sauce to cut back on the fat content and so that you can enjoy the flavor of the pasta.
- **Experiment with whole grain pastas,** which contain twice the fiber, and which will keep you fuller longer.
- **Remember the words of La Signora: pasta doesn't make people fat.** The same can be said for pizza. It's not pizza that makes a person fat. It's what you put on top of it and how much you eat. A reasonably-sized slice once in a while isn't going to hurt you if you're careful about the toppings. Eat it with a fresh salad and maybe round it out with a digestion-enhancing glass of wine.
- **And if at some point you absolutely have to snack, try a few pieces of leftover pasta.** And *basta*! That should tide you over.

Chapter 6:

Principles of Eating Italian Style

He who eats well, lives well.
—Italian proverb

Italian food is comforting, substantial, *and* sticks to your ribs. But as you're learning, it can fill you up, but it doesn't have to fill you out.

When you eat Italian style, you can finally say goodbye to neurotic dieting behavior that makes your life miserable and doesn't lead to lasting weight loss, anyway. There's no sense of deprivation because you eat well. You just limit your eating to three meals a day in appropriate proportions—with an occasional small snack, because Italians like to feel that they can break rules.

Weight loss, Italian style is not a fad. It's about getting back to the common sense you lost somewhere along the way—probably because it's not taught in schools and is certainly not demonstrated in the majority of American families. (And don't get me started on what Madison Avenue and the advertising world does!)

Don't Diet—Live!

I'm not going to bore you with a bunch of technical stuff. I don't enjoy technical diet books. They overwhelm me. I don't like counting calories or getting on bathroom scales, either. They drive me crazy. I'd rather do something natural, like just enjoy my food and my life. Eating is not a problem as long as we follow some simple guidelines. Like those contained in the following Latin proverb, (also attributed to seventeenth century clergyman Thomas Fuller):

Eat well, drink in moderation, and sleep sound.
In these three, good health abounds.

The Italian way of eating is to eat well, in a way that's healthy, satisfying, and sane. It's about feeling satiated by delicious, flavorful food that's prepared simply and eaten under the right circumstances, in appropriate portions. It's about putting food back into its proper perspective so that you can live a life not dominated by dieting and weight issues.

We're talking about exchanging quantity for quality—eating less but making it better and more satisfying. The Italian secret is to enjoy great food within limits rather than mediocre junk piled high on a plate—or out of a bag or carton.

But isn't limiting consumption the problem of everyone who wants to lose weight? Isn't that what you fear the most? You think it's going to be painful and you're going to starve. It's my contention that if you start eating the kinds of foods that really fulfill your body's needs, you'll be satisfied with less than when you graze or stuff yourself with junk food, or when you starve, then stuff. Good food in proper proportion, as opposed to junk food, is restorative for the body. It even helps your mind. Eating a robust, healthy diet really will put a brake on your desire to snack. I know, because I've tried it, and it works.

Now it's your turn to create this for yourself. There's a refined joy in learning a new way of being—in feeling good about your choices and knowing you can trust yourself not to be hijacked by visions of cupcakes, sugarplums, or whatever it is that thwarts you and destroys your resolve. Giving in to desires never gets rid of them. They're immediately replaced by new desires. Good habits are so much more satisfying in the long run. They're your invisible food chastity belt.

It's really about creating a new relationship with food. Eat sumptuous foods in smaller quantities. Save up for the banquet. Don't eat the slop. You won't miss the quantity because the quality is so much better.

Dieting is not living. Counting calories can become an obsession that sucks the joy out of eating. If you've lost your sense of what a normal portion is, you may need to count calories in the beginning, if that's what you do now. But by retraining your food monitor, your goal is to reach the point where you know just by looking at food what's right for you and how much to eat. There was a time in your life when you could do this. Your body has a memory of what that was like and would really appreciate a return to it.

The Seventeen Principles of Pleasurable Weight Loss

Yes, you will probably have to eat less if you want to lose weight. But that doesn't mean you have to starve or feel deprived. Quite the contrary. When you eat Italian style, you will be eating better and will feel more satisfied. So I'd like to share seventeen simple principles to follow to help you start eating and living in a way that supports your weight loss and maintenance. You don't have to memorize them. Just hold them loosely in your head.

There's a printer-friendly version at www.WeightLossItalianStyle. com/jillspantry. You can print out a copy and hang it on your refrigerator to glance at during the day—or before you open the fridge. Once you know the principles, the rest is easy. You can't make a mistake! So let me lay out these seventeen foundational principles in a list, and then we can go more deeply into detail:

1. Make eating an experience.
2. Engage the senses.

3. Good food in proper proportion.
4. Eat like a gourmet, not a glutton.
5. Use the replacement army.
6. *Piano! Piano!* (Slow down!)
7. Eat in courses.
8. Eliminate snacking, the Great American Diet Downfall.
9. Get rid of junk food.
10. Don't eat anything bigger than your fist.
11. Hunger is the best spice.
12. Eat well, and don't skip meals.
13. Wind down with a little wine.
14. Eat with the seasons.
15. Fall in love with olive oil.
16. Rely on basics.
17. Don't leave the chaperone at home!

Make Eating an Experience!

Don't eat—dine. What's the difference? It's the difference between lovemaking and a quickie. Dining implies that you're having an overall sensually satisfying experience, while eating suggests you're just filling your stomach with whatever you can get your hands on. When you dine instead of eat, it makes a tremendous difference in your relationship to food. Dining well is like living well. It's an act of self-love—even self-preservation. Italians dine, whereas Americans tend to eat ... and eat ... have a snack ... and then eat some more.

In Italy, eating is a joyous communal occasion, not something you do when you're home alone, stressed out, or unhappy in front of the television. It's not something you do just to distract yourself. A donut eaten standing up waiting for the bus is not breakfast, and a can of cola and a candy bar does not constitute dinner. For Italians, mealtime is life at its best, a convivial activity that nourishes both body and soul. Traditionally, it's a sacrosanct time when the family reconnects. It gives a person a sense of nourishment, contentment, and belonging. The companionship of loved ones—and the watchful eye of others—cushions the blows of the world and puts a brake on loneliness eating.

Unfortunately, the ritual of the family meal is going the way of the dinosaur in this country. But you can bring it back, or create your own variation of it by dining with others. There's value in ritual, especially this one. The Italians are right in making a big deal about breaking bread with loved ones and making mealtimes important occasions for connection. Studies have shown that teens that eat regular meals with their parents have better grades and run less risk of becoming depressed than their peers who don't eat with their families. Eating with others also gives adults a sense of community and makes them feel less vulnerable in the world at large.

Compared to the Italians, Americans tend to be loners. In Italy you don't see people eating by themselves the way you do in New York, for example. Their family ties are strong. I can remember staying with a family in Rome when a friend of theirs dropped by. They asked him to stay for dinner, but he couldn't because at forty years old, he still ate every meal with his mother. And if he didn't, there was trouble! Okay, this is going a little too far, but you get the picture. Eating together is important.

Many of us don't live anywhere near our families, let alone with them. And some of us don't have partners. If you're alone all the time there's a greater chance you'll feel depressed and eat too much. You may eat the wrong kinds of processed "comfort food" to soothe yourself.

Make your meals social occasions as often as possible. It's a quality of life issue. Learn how to cook and have people over, and maybe they'll do the same for you.

And even if you dine alone, make something exquisite and delicious. Set the table; pour yourself a nice glass of wine. Make it an event!

Engage the Senses

You don't have to eat staring at your kitchen wall or using the television for companionship. Eating in front of the television is a way to eat yourself fat. Don't stoop to mindlessly munching handfuls of junk out of a bag. Mealtime is the time to treat yourself like royalty. You don't have to go to a restaurant. A fine restaurant is great for a special occasion, but you can treat yourself right in the privacy of your own home. A well-stocked pantry, a pretty chandelier to hang over your table, a nice tablecloth and napkins can turn Casa You into the nicest restaurant in town.

This, of course, means giving up fast food, and that alone is cause for celebration. Not only is most fast food bad for you and full of things that can wreck your attempts to lose weight, the ambiance of a fast food restaurant is anything but restful. It's not conducive to good digestion or taking your time. Styrofoam cups, plastic silverware, cardboard dishes, and florescent lighting do not entice you to linger and enjoy your meal. The hard plastic seats and canned music make you want to scream and run.

I'm nothing if not realistic, and I know that sometimes fast food is the only game in town. But if you must pick up a commercially prepared meal, buy the most nutritious item on the menu you can find, and take it home and set a nice place for yourself.

If you have a garden, or even just a balcony, dine *al fresco* whenever possible. It's soothing to look upon grass, and flowers, and trees, and to hear birds singing. A garden setting is a fantastic setting for a meal. If you can't eat outside, create an inviting atmosphere inside your home that's conducive to the sensuous enjoyment of food.

Be the guest at your own table. Cover it with a tablecloth. Use candles and pretty napkins and your most appealing dishes. This is not kindergarten. No plastic plates and placemats. Use the good stuff. Set a nice table. Put on some music and let Pavarotti or Andrea Bocelli serenade you in the background.

Engage *all* your senses, so your stomach isn't running the show.

Treat food like sex. A glass of wine, antipasto, and conversation are the foreplay that creates anticipation and excitement for the main course. It's better when you take your time. And don't forget to leave room for dessert.

Good Food in Proper Proportion

This is another way of saying, "Eat well at meals." In Italy, you don't eat all day long, and you don't just plop down any old thing on the table and call it food. It has to be good. You can reduce your weight and keep it down by eating delicious food three times a day. Keep it fresh, nutritious, and simple. And, like the Italians, have just enough food spread over just enough time for proper digestion to take place (at least ten to twenty minutes for each course, when possible).

At its most basic, eating Italian style is really about balance—creating a balance of freshness, simplicity, and flavor. By eating this way you leave the table feeling satisfied but not stuffed. It takes some effort to reverse years of eating and living the wrong way, but the resulting lifetime habit of healthy eating and weight maintenance will be worth it.

Eat Like a Gourmet, Not a Glutton

Italians love to eat, but they also like to look good. They're enthusiastic but disciplined eaters. No one wants to be perceived as a *mangione* (except maybe Chuck Mangione). They put a premium on style and wear pants with buttons and zippers, not elastic in the waist. Trim is in. They don't gorge like we do. Take their example and learn to appreciate good food and the feeling of contentment that follows eating just enough of it. It's the concept of "Just a little, but make it good."

I have a confession to make. I used to be a glutton. I found it hard to turn down sweets. However, after living in Italy, I learned to control my appetite and trained myself to want the right things—foods that taste good and do the double duty of nourishing my body. I've learned to become a disciplined eater. Why? Because I want to feel carefree and not have to think about it.

Pelegrino Artusi, the "father of Italian cooking," said that according to the Emperor Tiberius, by the age of thirty, a man should not need a doctor. Artusi took this to mean that by that age one should know how to eat properly, which really does diminish reasons to see a doctor. Gluttony sends people to the doctor. It "kills more than the sword."

Learn to appreciate the delectable taste of real food. Great food comforts and soothes you in a way that junk food can't. It pleases and delights you. But it's medicine more than entertainment.

Spend a little extra money on quality food. Eat less and eat better—sumptuous foods in smaller quantities. Savoring good food stretches the pleasure factor. Truly, less is more when you eat good food.

Here's a novel idea: eat when you're hungry. Stop before you're full. Not *when* you're full. Stop just a little before that. You don't have to stuff yourself. Pause as soon as you feel the first warmth of satisfaction in your stomach. Leave the table a little hungry. You won't be hungry for long, because your digestion will catch up with you twenty minutes later and tell you you've had enough. You won't starve, I promise! This is how you get your eating under control. Eat slowly, and then wait. Eventually this becomes your norm.

Then you can be a carefree eater.

Use the Replacement Army

Ripping out bad habits alone rarely works. The best, most lasting way to overcome bad habits is to replace them with good ones. I've heard this referred to as the "replacement army," because it's like having an army of support at your disposal. Don't say, "I'm going to stop using my car." It's too general. Say, "I'm going to walk to work instead of taking my car." Don't say, "I'm going to use the elevator less." Again, too general. Say, "I'm going to climb the stairs to my office three times this week." When you have a strategy and a replacement army to help you execute it, your life will become much nicer.

There's joy in learning a new way of being and feeling good about your choices and knowing that you can trust yourself. Don't just give up dessert. Learn to enjoy the juicy freshness of fruit instead. Don't just cut out processed food from your diet. Replace it with more nutritious, natural, and deeply satisfying items. Eat small amounts of delicious food, like cheese or even chocolate, rather than no-fat substitutes, which make you hungry later and tempt you into overeating.

Instead of starving on a lettuce salad, fortify yourself with fuel that lasts until the next meal. Like pasta, or better yet, a whole grain version. Eat a balanced diet of honest-to-goodness foods rather than junk and fake alternatives laden with chemicals.

Use the time you would normally use for snacking to do something else—something uplifting and beneficial, like taking a walk.

Piano, Piano! (Slow Down!)

This is what Italian girls learn to say to Italian boys, and although they're not talking about *food*, it's an appropriate phrase to introduce here. This is what Americans should learn to say to themselves. We eat so quickly we don't give ourselves enough time for a feeling of fullness and satisfaction to register before we're on to the next thing.

Give yourself time to decide whether or not you really need to continue eating. Take the time to check in with yourself. Learn to take stock with these questions:

- Do I really want anything else?
- Does continuing to eat benefit my body and my desire to lose weight?
- Would eating more just be a knee jerk reaction?
- How am I going to feel afterward? Pleased with myself or disappointed? Satisfied or stuffed?

If you wait long enough after you've eaten, you'll experience satiation. But the thing is, you have to stop eating *before* you feel full.

As I've said before, it takes twenty minutes for the signals between your brain and stomach to fully register. That's why eating in a hurry kills your weight loss efforts. So slow down. Savor every bite. Chew forty times. Have your appetizer or soup, wait ten to twenty minutes. Eat your next course. Wait ten or twenty minutes. In Italy, eating can last an hour—or two or three. There's food, and there's conversation. You probably don't have that much time, but relaxing over a meal when you can is restful—something we need to do as often as possible in our increasingly frenetic and overstressed existences.

Mind Your Manners Along With Your Weight

How can you make your meals more leisurely? You can start by practicing good table manners and waiting until everyone else is seated and served before you eat. You can stop multitasking. You don't need to be doing something else while you're eating. It's not a waste of time to just sit and relax and enjoy your meal. Turn off the TV, shut off your cell phone, and put down the book. All these activities detract from the dining experience and can cause you to lose track of how much you're eating.

If you're with others, enjoy their companionship. Have a face-to-face conversation instead of text messaging. The world won't stop. Notice what you're eating. How's the presentation? The color? How does it smell?

Ever heard the phrase, "Be here now"? Enjoy your food. Don't waste it by ruminating over the past or worrying about the future. If you're not in the present moment, you miss your life. And you miss your meal! Become present to eating and relishing food. Become a conscious eater. The price of going unconscious is obesity.

Eat in Courses

This is especially nice if the meal is punctuated by plenty of enlivening conversation. When a meal is divided into courses—the antipasto separate from the pasta, and the pasta separate from the meat, etc.—

you have plenty of time to feel your digestion catching up with your food intake. You'll be more likely to stop when you start feeling full. With courses, you don't proceed to the next item until the previous one has settled. Your meal takes longer, and by stretching things out, you may very well feel like passing up dessert. It's not a big deal to pass on sweets after a great meal. When you already feel satiated, you don't feel like you're missing out on anything.

Eating in courses definitely helps prevent Mindless Eating Syndrome where you just keep eating and eating without having any idea of how much you've eaten or how full you've become until it's too late. The Italian approach of a multicourse meal makes it seem as if you're eating more food. However, you may be consuming fewer calories in a four-course Italian meal than in one American dinner with everything piled high onto one plate.

If you can't eat in courses, at least serve items on separate plates. And clear the table before proceeding to your fruit.

Eliminate Snacking, the Great American Diet Downfall

Many women nibble their way to obesity without knowing how they got there. Be aware. Keep a record and be accountable to yourself. That's the only way to get control over your sticky fingers in the cupboard, fridge, and pantry. Eat well at meals, and don't keep snack food around the house.

People sometimes ask me, "Don't you ever feel like snacking?" For the most part, no, because I eat well at meals, so I don't get hungry in between. Occasions do arise—when I'm under a particular type of stress, for example—when I find myself going to the cupboard looking for something to eat. But I usually don't find it because I don't keep snack food on hand.

What do I do in that case? I have a piece of apple with a little bit of cheese (to slow down the digestive process), or a small handful of nuts. Or a few pieces of leftover whole grain pasta. Or a little serving of beans drizzled with olive oil and a sprinkle of salt. Or a small piece of bread dipped in olive oil. It's never regular snack food—that's too dangerous. It's just a little something made of what's already in the kitchen.

Eating a robust, healthy diet based on grains, olive oil, fruits and vegetables, and small amounts of lean meat will curb your desire for the Great American Diet Downfall—between-meal snacking. Spend at least a week logging every time you put something in your mouth: when you eat, what and how much you eat, and what triggered the urge. After you get a look at your eating patterns, resolve to give up snacking by eating better at regular mealtimes by making better choices of foods that stay with you, such as pasta. Say goodbye to skimpy salads that don't fill you up and leave you vulnerable to late-afternoon munchies.

Counterattacks for Snacks

I don't believe in snacking. I just don't. Your digestive system deserves a rest once in a while, and you won't enjoy your meals as much if you ruin your appetite. Chronic snackers don't lose weight. A snack once in a while won't hurt, but the problem is that people who like to snack make "once in a while" habitual, and this can destroy your efforts.

Eat well at mealtimes and choose quality foods, not junk food or low-fat, fake versions of food. Skip the snack foods and drinks when you go to a movie. Walk right by the snack counter and go to your seat. Do it with the right mindset. Be *glad* you're not snacking because you're looking forward to a good meal afterward or have already enjoyed a leisurely, luxurious Italian-style feast beforehand.

Be like those Italians I met on Elba. Or La Signora in Florence. Focus on what you're going to have for dinner that night. Allow yourself to long for it and fantasize about it. Make it something good that you can look forward to. Think about how satisfying it's going to be and don't ruin it by eating between meals. Save your calories for an enjoyable meal in the evening when you can relax at the end of the day, preferably with good company. Fantasize! Anticipate! And don't kill the thrill of satiating your hunger by snacking before the main meal.

If you don't plan ahead, your hunger may derail you. If you decide on the spur of the moment when you're hungry, you may not make the best meal choice.

My biggest weaknesses were always desserts and junk food. Learning to eat the Italian way allowed me to let go of the hold that these foods had on me and still feel satisfied—to the point that I lost my craving for them. Now I never crave these foods. I may eat birthday cake or a dessert on special occasions, but I'm never tempted to go out of my way to eat them. I'm rarely tempted to eat badly, because eating well is so satisfying. I never feel crazy or possessed by the need to have something. Knowing the misery of food cravings and the havoc they can play in your life, I'm grateful to the Italians for teaching me to enjoy the flavor of good, delicious food, simply prepared, eaten under the right circumstances, and in appropriate proportions.

And when you eat well, you can break the rules once in a while.

Get Rid of Junk Food

Dig new ditches. Wean yourself off sweets and snacks. Junk food has to become a thing of the past. Be happy about this. It means you're taking care of yourself. Hopefully you'll go through the kitchen and dump the junk. Don't be sentimental. Don't think of the money you've wasted. Just get rid of it. The life you save, and certainly the waistline, may be your own.

What is junk food? For me, the definition is a lot like the one they use for pornography: I can't tell you what it is exactly, but I know it when I see it! If you have any doubt as to what constitutes junk food, read the labels. If it sounds like a science experiment, toss it.

If you think no one lives in a kitchen without junk food or processed food, let me describe to you what I discovered one morning while sitting in La Signora's kitchen in Florence. She always left coffee warming for me in the mornings when she'd be off on her bike fetching fresh items for dinner that night.

I remember looking around the kitchen as I was drinking my coffee and wondering what kind of food an Italian cooking teacher kept on hand. Was I ever shocked when the only things I could find were dried pasta, olive oil, vinegar, salt and pepper, some fresh fruit, and coffee. Her tiny refrigerator was empty, and she had no freezer. There was practically no shelf space. She didn't need it because she ate everything fresh and shopped daily and used everything she bought. There was nothing to raid in her kitchen even if I'd wanted to.

This surprises many Americans. My friend Dirk, who was stationed in the Navy in Gaeta, ran into a similar situation while staying with his Italian girlfriend's (now his wife's) family. He happened to look in the refrigerator and saw it was empty. He thought the family was hurting and that maybe he'd better start chipping in for meals. Actually, they were one of the prominent families in their village. What he didn't realize was that the fridge was empty because the father shopped for fresh food every day—on foot. That's how he stayed healthy.

Once you get used to eating the fresh and healthy Italian way, you're not going to miss your processed junk food, especially the low-fat, no-fat items you thought were saving you from hunger and feelings of deprivation.

Don't Eat Anything Bigger Than Your Fist

This is a good rule of thumb, though of course it can't be taken literally all the time. But you can think about it when you look at your plate. Take small servings—a small piece of meat, only one or two pieces of bread, and a small dessert. You can afford to eat sumptuous foods if they're in small quantities.

In our culture, people have come to expect large portions and oversized everything and feel cheated if they don't get them. Italian portions are smaller. Coffee comes in the size of what we'd associate with a teacup, and you don't get seconds. An espresso cup hardly holds an egg. A cup of coffee we once ordered on the train was the size of a free sample coffee you get at some grocery stores in the States. Over there, it's not considered skimpy. They're just accustomed to smaller portions.

Your choice of dishes is important, too. Use a smaller plate and your small portion will appear larger. It will trick your mind into thinking you're eating a lot. Brian Wansink of Cornell University, the snacking expert and author of *Mindless Eating: Why We Eat More Than We Think*, suggests that the size of a plate, bowl, or container of food profoundly affects how much a person eats. In one of his more notable experiments, participants were fed a substantial lunch and then invited to a movie where they were given different-sized buckets of popcorn. Despite the fact that the popcorn was stale and practically inedible, people given the largest buckets ate up to 34 percent more popcorn than those given smaller containers.

I had an experience kind of like this, recently. I was at a restaurant where I was served the equivalent of three portions of chicken piccata (one-and-a-half chicken breasts) on a plate that was about twelve inches in diameter. The serving was huge. In Italy, half of one of those gigantic breasts would be considered a meal, but it didn't look that way on the plate. So I ended up cleaning my plate rather than checking in with my stomach, because it didn't look like a lot of food. The large plate size tripped me up.

This is true for beverages, too. Soft drinks at restaurants in Italy come in small, expensive glasses, and you don't get seconds. Since you know that, you savor what you have and gauge your intake to make it last throughout the meal. Italians eat and drink in quantities vaguely reminiscent of how it used to be in America—*before* our obesity crisis.

Hunger is the Best Spice

Mild, occasional feelings of hunger are nothing to fear and should not send you into a tailspin. They're normal. You're supposed to feel hungry before you eat a meal. Mild hunger pangs are the "spice" that increases your enjoyment of food.

Learn to embrace this paradox. Restrain yourself until mealtimes to heighten the enjoyment of eating. Pull back and deny yourself a little, then enjoy fully. Eat slowly. The experience will be exquisite.

Eat Well, and Don't Skip Meals

Eat well at every meal. Don't try to skip breakfast. It won't give you the outcome you desire. You'll get hungry and be tempted to snack. According to a study published in the *American Journal of Clinical Nutrition* in February 2005, skipping breakfast can lead to weight gain. In the study, healthy women who skipped breakfast were seen to eat more during the course of the day than those who ate breakfast. And a study of Northern Italian children that same year showed higher rates of obesity in those who skipped breakfast compared to those who didn't.

Breakfast in Italy, or *colazione*, tends to be a light meal of some kind of coffee—espresso, cappuccino or caffe latte—with a roll, bread, or a small pastry. To give you an idea of just how small "small" can be, I was once at someone's house and was given a thimble of espresso and two tiny cookies before we set out on an all-day drive around Lake Como. I looked at it and thought, *You've got to be kidding!* But it made lunch at a nice restaurant later all the more pleasurable. Fresh fish from the lake never tasted so good.

Your breakfast doesn't have to be this small! You could eat some fruit and add a little peanut butter or an egg to your bread to help keep you from getting hungry later. The main function of *colazione* is to keep you going until the more substantial lunch at midday, not so many hours away.

Most Italians used to eat their lunch, or *pranzo*, with the family. In more traditional areas, lunch is still a family affair, with both a first and second course. During my stays in Italy, *pranzo* was followed by a rest before people went back to work at 4:00 PM. This no longer holds true in big cities where, like here, many now have to grab a quick panino and get back to the office. Dinner has become the family gathering time.

If you can swing it, an ideal lunch would be a small serving of pasta with a small serving of meat, salad, and a little vegetable. Or you could have pasta with a salad and a piece of fruit to follow if you're still hungry. Lighter fare would be a frittata (or omelet) with soup or salad. You could also have just a hearty soup or a rice dish like risotto with a green salad.

I always make myself a good lunch, and it doesn't take much time, even though I never use a microwave. I make pasta, gnocchi, a frittata or a *caprese* salad with tomatoes, basil, and fresh mozzarella. I have to move around my kitchen to do it and go outside to collect fresh herbs, so I get a little exercise while I'm at it. It's a joyful activity.

Dinner could be something similar, perhaps cutting back on the starchy items and adding a lean protein course, with fruit for dessert. For dinner you might have a salad, a small amount of pasta with a lean protein and a vegetable, followed by fruit and coffee. Wine makes the meal more pleasant and stimulates conversation. Meat and fish can be alternated with bean dishes. The Italians are not big meat eaters and often meet their protein requirements by eating beans and other legumes.

Get into the habit of eating fruit rather than a sugary dessert. In Italy, fruit follows the meal. Eat sweets sparingly, maybe on Saturday night or with a Sunday dinner. If you keep desserts small and reserve them for special occasions, they can still have a place in your life. And you don't have to feel guilty about it.

But I do mean small. The strawberry mousse recipe that I obtained from Academia Barilla, (which is in your bonus recipe download) considers that you're making servings about the size of a mini muffin. It's rich, so that's all you need at the end of a meal. In America, we're brainwashed into thinking we need something bigger. But look where it's brought us. Take a tip from the Italians and from fine restaurants and keep your desserts small. Eat them slowly, and savor every bite.

Most Italians I know eat bread with their meal. If you're eating pasta or gnocchi and watching your weight, you should probably skip the bread. Use your judgment and see what works best for you. If a little bread satisfies you so that you don't want to snack later, indulge yourself. However, if you see that you're having trouble getting your weight to budge, you may have to substitute bread for pasta rather than eat them at the same time.

On special occasions, you might even want to finish off your dinner Italian style with a coffee "corrected" by a shot of grappa. Or have a sip of *limoncello*. (Not in your coffee!) It's a delicious and very potent liqueur made with fresh lemons.

Wind Down with a Little Wine

Wine is a part of Italian habit, life, and culture. Having wine with dinner is not only normal in Italy, it's expected. It enhances the taste of food and does not carry the stigma it sometimes does in the States. In America we're told that wine adds calories. But many Italians feel that wine enjoyed with a meal burns calories. Odd as it appears, this has seemed to be my experience. How do you account for that, considering that a glass of wine contains about eighty calories? Probably because it aids digestion when drunk in moderation—say, a glass or two with a meal.

"Food and wine always go together," Bette Ann Bierwirth of Antinori, maker of some of Italy's most highly regarded wines, told me when I visited their estates outside of Florence. In fact, she said, "Wine is liquid food." It helps Italians relax when they come home from work in the evening. "They even sip wine while fixing a meal and it makes the food taste better! You don't have to drink much."

An Italian friend of mine insists that dinner always starts with a glass of wine, "five or ten minutes before Mamma serves the spaghetti."

Ms. Bierwirth praised wine's ability to bring out the best even in modest foods. "The combination of simple pecorino cheese with wine is paradise. Or bread with olive oil. It's a dream come true, a pleasure. For us, wine is history, art, and food. It's part of the big picture of eating. It *is* history. It has been made forever and ever."

Pairing wine with food is an art. I'm sure you know the basic: red wine with meat and white wine with fish or fowl. "Except," Maurizio Colia, sommelier at Osteria di Passignano, an Antinori-owned restaurant and cooking school in the Chianti region, told me, "for pinot noir, which is the only red wine that goes with fish." He said it's a fantastic companion to cheese.

The considerations regarding wine become more complex depending on the richness of the food and its intensity. You don't want the wine to overpower the food or vice versa. It's a balancing act.

Eat with the Seasons

Eating with the seasons means eating what's best for you and what tastes best also. Think of a fresh peach. It doesn't even need sugar. How can you improve upon perfection? Nature's bounty is ours to enjoy, and seasonal foods are key to Italian-style eating.

Eating seasonally is a beautiful, nurturing, and satisfying way of increasing your enjoyment of food. I remember being served fresh ripened figs for dessert one time on Elba in August. No fancy dessert could have compared with them. They were perfect. Eating with the seasons is a sensual pleasure that can heighten your appreciation of the locally grown produce. It means eating what's best for you when it tastes the best.

Whenever possible, be like the Italians and eat what's in season. I know we used to think, "Oh boy, strawberries in December!" when we would see imported fruits in the dead of winter. The problem was, they really didn't taste like strawberries. Or not like the summer strawberries I remembered. So, out-of-season fruits may be nice for a special occasion, but it's really more satisfying to eat them when they arrive in summer. And here's a food equation I live by:

Anticipation + delayed gratification = ultimate satisfaction

Fall in Love with Olive Oil

I began my love affair with olive oil in Rome on a hot day in June many years ago. I had just arrived from America, I didn't speak a word of Italian, and I was starving. It was past the regular lunch hour, so most places were closed. I finally found a place that seemed to be open and mustered up the courage to go inside and try to order some lunch. The first thing the waiter brought me was a bowl of soup with globules of oil swimming on the top. It looked weird, and I thought I had chosen the wrong restaurant. But I was ravenous and decided that something was better than nothing. I lifted my spoon to take a mouthful, but before I did, a fragrant aroma hit my nose. It was rich, and herby, and delicious. Needless to say, so was the soup.

Next came an omelet. It was the first time I'd ever had an omelet cooked in olive oil, and it was the last time I ever made my own with butter. Olive oil became a part of my life. Now I use olive oil on everything, because the sharp, distinctive flavor of high-quality extra virgin olive oil has me hooked. I use olive oil instead of mayonnaise and butter. I even use it on toast with a sprinkle of salt.

Given the choice between eating extra virgin olive oil for the rest of my life or chocolate, olive oil would win hands down. It's delicious, full of antioxidants and high in monosaturated fats, which can lower the risk of heart disease. (Yes, I know that dark chocolate has antioxidant properties, but a person shouldn't really eat sweets morning, noon, and night!)

Olive oil enhances the delectable flavor of food. I can go into ecstasy over olive oil. But you must use extra virgin. It's the least processed and the most tasty and healthful. It has the highest level of polyphenols.

Many Italians flavor their salads with nothing but olive oil and a little salt. I've started doing this, too, because it's more healthy and, in my opinion, tastier than commercial dressings.

To truly appreciate olive oil, I suggest that for dressing salads and for drizzling on food, you experiment with the more expensive artisan brands. I particularly like the peppery flavor of Tuscan olive oils. They wake up your taste buds and give your food an unmistakable "That's Italian!" flavor.

Rely on Basics

Few things are as annoying as setting out to make something for dinner and realizing that you're lacking a particular ingredient. When I used to cook all types of food, this happened all the time. Now that I focus on Italian food, I can always make something good based on what's already in my kitchen. Shopping, too, has become a breeze. You can actually shop in your head without using a list for most things and your cupboard never needs to be bare.

While we're sharing the secrets of Italy, let me tell you the secret of shopping like an Italian. All you have to do is picture the Italian flag: red, white, and green. Those are the colors of Italian food and a reminder of the kitchen basics you should never be without. Red is for tomatoes and red peppers. White is for garlic, parmesan (parmigiano-reggiano is best), pasta, and mozzarella. And green is for extra virgin olive oil and fresh basil.

Just remember that when you do your shopping and you'll always have the makings of something tasty. Or you can use this fun, silly memory device that I learned from an Italian friend:

- Right hand (absolute musts): dried pasta, olive oil, garlic, tomatoes, parmigiano-reggiano cheese
- Left hand (runners up): basil, capers, tomato paste, anchovies, wine
- Right foot (useful and tasty): cannellini beans, onions, red pepper flakes, packaged gnocchi, olives
- Left foot (you shouldn't even have to think about these): fresh fruit, fresh vegetables, coffee, sparkling mineral water, bread

See how easy?

Cooking Italian style makes life simple. Otherwise I wouldn't do it. When you have these things around, you're always able to whip up something that tastes good.

Don't Leave the Chaperone at Home

Along with your wallet, valid ID, hairbrush, lipstick, and mints, you need to take your inner chaperone with you wherever you go—including into your own kitchen.

Who is this chaperone who will gently but firmly guide you to the right choices? It's your "inner thinner"—the slimmer person that's inside you who wants to be reflected on the outside. If you follow all the above guidelines, you'll automatically be behaving like a thin person. But you need to think like one, too. Your "inner thinner" is there to jog the part of your mind that knows that's what you are —a thin person temporarily occupying a body that's a little larger than you'd like. But at heart you are a thin person who naturally thinks in a thin way.

Stay in character and act the part. In America, we say fake it until you make it. In Italy, if they said it, it would be something like, *Imbroglia fino a che ci riesci!*

Your Action Plan—Steps You Can Take *Now*

You learned a lot in this chapter, and now it's time to put some of the most important strategies into practice. The first step is to go to www.WeightLossItalianStyle.com/jillspantry and print out the list of "Seventeen Principles of Pleasurable Weight Loss." Hang it on your refrigerator and refer to it often until the principles are second nature. Also, download your "Bad Habit/Replacement Army" worksheet and fill it out. Carry it in your pocket to refer to in emergency food situations.

The second step is to memorize the Italian flag colors (red, white, green) and what they represent in food choices. And if you wish, you can consider learning my friend's "fingers and toes" shopping strategy. Also:

- Make meals a celebration by eating with other people when possible.
- Feed yourself through your senses and not just your mouth.
- Focus on what you eat. Contemplate it. Savor it. Fall in love with each bite.
- Go out and buy a small amount of your favorite food and enjoy it.

Chapter 7:

Managing Your Mind— the Real Alchemy

Pluck the rose and leave the thorns.
—Italian proverb

If you ever wanted to give up on yourself or if it's seemed impossible to develop the discipline necessary for losing weight and keeping it off, the answer is closer than you think. It's not in your own two hands. It's between your ears. Your struggle is more with your mind than your body.

The mind is very tricky. It makes a great slave but a terrible master. Most of us are walking around as slaves to unruly, self-defeating thoughts, and we don't even know it. An untamed mind is like a pair of runaway Roman chariot horses. You can't control them, and they take you places you don't want to go. That horsepower of your unruly mind drags you to the refrigerator ... and your cupboards ... and the cookie aisle and ice cream sections of stores.

Maybe sometimes you get an inkling of this. Have you ever felt like a *schiava*, or slave, to food? Don't tell me. I already know.

So the big question is: how do you go from being the *schiava* to being the *maestra*?

Why Master the Mind?

Particularly where weight loss is concerned, we become overly focused on our physical body when the mind is the key to everything. It's the guts of your entire being and definitely "the boss of you" unless you are the boss of it. Your mind decides what to eat and when. Your mind decides whether you're going to exercise or sit on the couch and watch TV. Your body is just a slave to your thoughts, but we treat the body as if it's the mastermind behind the crime when we overeat. Poor body!

Trying to change behavior when the mind is not willing is painful, if not impossible. One of the main reasons why dieting hasn't worked for you is probably because you've been trying to *control your behavior without changing your mind*. If your body changes but you continue to obsess about food, the chances are that you'll be like more than 90 percent of those who lose weight, and you won't be able to keep it off permanently.

Your mind is your "big gun" in the war on obesity. How you use it is even more important than what you eat or how much you exercise, because your mind controls both of these behaviors. Fortunately, you can learn to control your mind. It is, in fact, the only thing you have any real control over, but very few people exercise this power.

Your Mind Is your Genie

The ancient Romans believed that every person had an unseen guide or "genius" (*iuno*, for women) that helped them navigate through life. Actually, they weren't far from the truth. Your mind is not only your genius; it acts as your personal genie. How? Because in a very real sense it grants your wish by attracting into your life whatever you focus upon. We experience the world based on our habitual thoughts. If you choose thoughts of excess weight, you will experience the world through that lens. If you choose uplifting thoughts, that's what your world reflects. It all depends on how you see things.

Masters of the mind say that what we think about is projected outward onto the screen of the world much the way a movie is projected from a machine onto a screen. This is why I urge you to *think of yourself as a person who is becoming slender* rather than one who is overweight. Otherwise you may find yourself sitting through a very long, bad movie that would seem to be not of your choice—except that it is.

Be conscious of what you're thinking about from moment to moment, because your thoughts set the stage for what you experience. If you feel critical of yourself or your body, you're just reinforcing what you don't want.

If you're like many people, you probably don't give much thought to where your thoughts come from or how much they affect you, but according to a little book called *The Kybalion* (first published in December 1908), your thought is the greatest natural force in the material world.

The teachings of this book are based upon ancient hermeticism, which found its way to Italy through works translated by the Medici Court and which were said to help fuel the Renaissance. (Some of the teachings are consistent with New Age thought, but they're actually "Age Old.") The foundational principal that "all is mind" tells us that the universe is a mental construct. Everything we see and experience— you, me, our physical, mental, and dream worlds—may be thought of as one intelligent, living, universal mind that creates mentally, using nothing outside of itself.

Your mind is part of this. It was created by this universal mind, but you also create your own worlds by the way you think. And then you live in your creation. Isn't your world, or more accurately, your *experience* of the world, different than your neighbor's or a member of your family's, even though you live in the same house? Have you ever gone to a movie with a friend and loved it while they hated it? Same movie, different opinion.

Or have you ever thought ahead to an event that hasn't yet taken place? You enact everything in your mind, including whom you're going to see, what you're going to say to them, and what they say back. You may even start to upset yourself because of what you imagine is taking place in this world you've created. And it isn't even real.

If you start really paying attention to your thoughts, you'll see how often you bring yourself down with negative, self-defeating ones. Being negative toward anything keeps you in the cycle of remaining unhappy, which leads to overeating. It may seem hard to reverse a lifetime of ingrained negative thinking patterns, but it's not impossible.

Be Vigilant

The biggest hurdle here, and it is a big one, is staying aware of when you do this. You need to make an effort to uplift yourself on a continuous basis. Be like the Italians, who are a congenial people and who like to keep things upbeat. (Think of the music of Rossini, or, again, the movies of Roberto Benigni.) In general, Italians make an effort to be happy and to experience pleasure. If you wallow in negative thoughts, you experience life through a negative veil. If you choose positive thoughts, you experience a pleasant world. We really do create our own reality from moment to moment based on what we think about. If you believe something, then it's true for you.

Even whether you have a good day or a lousy day depends less on what happened than on how you perceive it. Good and bad are relative. When you think about your weight, you have a choice of making yourself depressed by how many pounds you believe you need to lose or uplifting yourself by telling yourself how great it is that you're finally losing the weight. You decide what spin you put on the situation. Is the cappuccino cup half empty or half full? It depends on how you look at it, not on how much you've drunk.

We all know that you're more vulnerable to binging when you're feeling down. But you don't have to be a victim of your moods. You can change your mind as easily as you can talk to a friend in Rome by pressing a few buttons on your phone. We think nothing of performing such "miracles" numerous times a day without even thinking of it. But change our mind? *Mamma mia!* Are you *pazza* (crazy)?

And yet we know from experience that it's possible to change our minds, because we do it all the time. Think of an occasion when you were feeling bad and suddenly you received a phone call that uplifted you. We have the ability to go from sad to happy in an instant, but we usually don't exercise this power on our own. We let circumstances do it for us.

You've Got the Power

Remember the next time you're gripped by the desire to snack that *you have the power to change your mind.* Do whatever it takes to change the channel. Play some upbeat Italian accordion music, dance, or call a friend. Take a walk. You can even practice your Italian on the people you run across— *"Ciao!" "Buon giorno!" (*Rent the movie, *Breaking Away*, and see how it's done.)

Nothing bad is going to happen if you postpone your trip to the kitchen. If you don't dig into those biscotti today, trust me; they'll still be there tomorrow. Just by postponing your desire you may be able to short-circuit the need to eat. Then postpone it a little longer. By tomorrow, or even fifteen minutes later, you may have forgotten about them.

Newsflash—Your Weight Is *Not* Permanent

The only thing you can really count on in this world is change. Use this to your advantage the next time you find yourself depressed about your weight. Like everything else, it's a *temporary situation.* You're not stuck at the weight you think you are, because nothing stays the same. Everything is in a state of flux. That's why it's often a shock to run into someone you haven't seen in a number of years. They've changed.

You've probably experienced this scenario: you start a weight loss program, and at first you feel great. You're making so much progress, and then one day you make the mistake of stepping on the scale and see that you've gained a pound or two, and you feel like giving up. All that effort and this is what you get? Don't let it upset you. Everyone's weight fluctuates. Yours will change again if you stick with the process.

We think we can solve problems by dwelling on them, but usually the more you think about a problem, the more you stay stuck. What can you do instead? Just *shift the energy.* Go out and have fun. You don't need to get emotionally involved in what appears to be happening. Treat your inner struggle as if you're watching two people argue over the price of vegetables at the Campo dei Fiori. You don't need to get embroiled yourself. You can even choose to be amused by the display. Then go about your business.

You don't have control over everything that goes on in your life, but you have control over how you respond or interpret it. We get caught up in the fear that something unpleasant will stay with us forever when it's not necessarily the case. Instead of getting hysterical, maintain your composure like the Mona Lisa, who smiles secretly because she knows the inside joke that "this, too, shall pass." (I think she's also smiling because she's thinking about having pasta for dinner!) This is why I suggest staying away from the scale, because if you watch it too closely, it will drive you to despair. Better to watch the state of your mind. It's a better gauge of how you're doing.

Mood Swing

Opera's nice when you're sitting in the audience, but few of us can live peacefully with that much drama in real life. Do you go looking for it unintentionally?

There's a beautiful Italian proverb that counsels us to "Pluck the rose and leave the thorns." It's good advice.

Why condemn yourself to a bad mood when you can put yourself in a good one? I always think of a story told by an Italian friend of mine. One day she got in the car and set off for her job in Florence. Halfway there, she realized she'd forgotten something and had to turn around and go back home. But when she got there, she couldn't remember what she'd forgotten, which made things worse. On her way to her office, where she was going to arrive late, she came upon an accident involving many cars. And she realized that if she hadn't turned around and gone home she probably would have been in that accident.

You just never know. Better to try to find something to be thankful for, even when you think you have every reason to curse your fate. *Che sarà, sarà.* Whatever is meant to be, will be. And your life will seem much easier when you're no longer blown around at the mercy of every mood or feeling or change of plans. You really have a lot more control over your moods and feelings than you think, and you'll be surprised and delighted by the times you're able to master them.

Do you fall victim to overeating when you're feeling great or when you're feeling down? Most likely, when you're down. What kinds of thoughts are you entertaining at that time? Probably pessimistic ones. Until now you might not have noticed that pattern. You might even be so accustomed to it that you think it's normal.

In addition to changing the channel on your thoughts, what else can you do to change the pattern? You can short-circuit the desire to eat by *raising your vibration*. It's an actual physical thing, and the more attuned you become to your body, the more you'll feel the variations in vibe. It's like the lift you get from switching from some dismal dirge on one radio station to an upbeat song you like on another.

That's actually one way of raising your vibration with outside help. Bouncy music lifts you. Buy some jaunty Italian mandolin or accordion music and play it when you feel yourself sliding into a funk. You can also raise your vibe by dancing, taking a walk or a drive, riding a bicycle, singing, kissing, or making love. Just get your energy moving in a different direction.

What do you like to do? Drop what you're doing and do it. You know what makes you happy. You just have to push through that irksome resistance and self-indulgent desire to wallow when you could lift yourself. We fall victim to that desire sometimes, because we secretly think it will bring us what we want. But it never does. Usually it makes things worse. Instead, change your energy. Flip the switch on your feeling, not just your thought.

Do it with the strength of your mind.

It doesn't matter how unsuccessful you've been in the past. If you develop the right frame of mind, you can achieve your weight loss goals. A winning mindset leaves no room for failure.

Napoleon Hill, author of the classic *Think and Grow Rich* (first published by The Ralston Society in 1938), said, "Whatever the mind can conceive and believe, the mind can achieve." Hill was coached by steel magnate and philanthropist Andrew Carnegie, who told him that everyone comes to this planet with the equivalent of two sealed envelopes—one filled with the riches they will enjoy if they take possession of their mind and the other filled with penalties if they don't. The "riches" bag contained good health, freedom from fear, and material riches, among other things. The "penalties" bag contained everything undesirable. Hill made it his mission to teach people how to access and use the "riches" bag. His instruction? Buy a notebook and write down a clear description of your big desire. Write down also what you will give in return for the fulfillment of that desire, and then start giving it immediately. He said to write down and memorize both statements and to repeat them to yourself twelve times every day.

His next instruction was very interesting. He said that each repetition should be followed by a statement of gratitude asking not for more riches, but for the wisdom to use what you already have—the power to harness your mind toward whatever you want.

Why are his instructions powerful? They focus your mind upon a desired outcome so that there's little room for doubts or fears or backsliding. Everything in your life starts funneling toward the picture of what you want, because there's no provision for anything else. You put your mind to work as your servant, which is a whole lot better than the other way around. Like Christopher Columbus and Amerigo Vespucci (the first from Genoa, the second from Florence), you become captain of your ship rather than a lowly stowaway.

If you're focused on your goal, you won't drift off course, even in the face of temptation—like when your Italian neighbor comes around with a batch of cannoli. You can take just one and pass the rest around to your crew.

The bottom line is this: become master of your mind. Don't give energy to any mental image of yourself as overweight or any negative feelings about your life, because that only reinforces it. Raise your vibration. Accentuate the positive. Put your attention onto the woman you are becoming. Start acting the part, and let it be reflected in the clothes you wear, the way you hold yourself, and the food you eat.

If you develop the right frame of mind, you can achieve your weight loss goals. A winning mindset leaves no room for failure.

Your Action Plan—Steps You Can Take *Now*

- Make yourself a bold weight loss goal.
- Write it down.

To reinforce your lowered weight, on paper you may want to create your own weight loss "thermometer." Just draw a thermometer like the kind you hang outside your house to keep track of the temperature. Write your current weight at the top and your ideal weight at the bottom. (Make sure it's a weight you believe is attainable.)

Tape the paper to your bathroom mirror and refer to it as often as possible. You could also create a version for your pocket.

- "See" your weight at the number you desire on the thermometer.
- Make it so real for yourself that you can feel it in the cells of your body.
- Refer to it several times a day.

Chapter 8:

Activate Your Passion!

There is no end. There is no beginning.
There is only the infinite passion of life.
—Federico Fellini.

Italian culture is infused with passion. It drives Italian relationships, Italian cuisine and dining, the way Italians converse, and especially the way they make love!

Walk into a restaurant in any part of the world, and you know which table the Italians are occupying. Everyone's talking with their hands as well as their mouths. Enter a Roman piazza after sundown, and you'll see passion in full swing, in the laughter of revelers spilling onto the sidewalks from cafes, in the roar of the scooters zooming around corners, and in the intent gazes of couples engaging in *la passagiata*, sitting on statues, necking and falling in love.

Italians come by their passion honestly. Their forerunners were, for lack of a better word, pagans. In some ways Italians still are. Their gregarious pursuit of happiness is one of their charms. Ancient Italians believed in energies or natural forces that influenced everything, from household prosperity to a woman's menstruation and a man's ejaculation. Later they gave these divine energies human forms and built temples to them up and down the peninsula. You can still visit the ruins of temples to the Mother Goddess, Isis, and her various aspects as Vesta, Venus, Juno, Minerva, and others. Some of these temples reorganized as churches to Mary when Christianity took over.

Pagan passions carried over in a more acceptable form to the 1950s and 1960s when Italy spawned voluptuous stars, or so-called sex goddesses, such as Sophia Loren, Gina Lollobrigida, and Claudia Cardinale—back in the days when it was okay to have curves and a light-hearted hedonism was considered a good thing.

Who can argue with the desire to seek pleasure and avoid pain, as long as it doesn't hurt you or anyone else? In fact, acknowledging your own pagan passion—what could be referred to as your "goddess energy"—can assist your weight loss process, since it's really about reconnecting with and relishing your wholeness. The more you access and embody the earthy, outrageous, playful, intelligent, and elegant part of you, the better you'll feel about yourself and the rest of your life. (The less whole you feel, the more you're going to try to fill the gaps with food.)

Goddesses are part of our world whether we acknowledge them or not. A big, imposing goddess sits in New York Harbor, attracting millions of visitors each year. (You probably know her as the Statue of Liberty.) Another graces the top of the Capitol building in Washington, D.C. We even have our own American goddess, "Columbia." And if you decorate your Thanksgiving table with a cornucopia, you're honoring Isis. (It's her symbol of *abbondanza*.) Goddesses are here; goddesses are there. Goddesses are everywhere, if you just start noticing. We can learn from what they represent: our best, and in some cases disowned, qualities. (When you get really good at it, you may even find one staring back at you from your bathroom mirror.)

You're something deeper than all the likes and dislikes that make up your personality. You have intuition and *blunted sources of power*. And part of the pain you feel—the part of it that drives you to overeating—is the pain of not expressing those untapped parts of yourself. Uncovering them is as exciting as digging through rubble down to uncover a buried treasure, like your own Pompeii. So get out your archeological tools. We're going to do some excavating. As some wise teacher told one of my teachers, who passed it on to me, "The problem is not that life is so short. It's that we've been dead so long."

Start living.

Playtime for Your Inner Goddess

Invite your inner goddess to come out and play. By honoring goddesses on the outside, Roman women were able to connect with the goddessy parts of themselves on the inside—their passionate, loving, energetic nature. If you're always hungry, consider that what you may be hungry for is your own fun-filled spirit. We're all walking repositories of passion, but few of us get to experience this.

Trust your instincts. Contact with your goddess aspect helps you gather up the disparate parts of yourself and love yourself back to health and harmony. You need only three things on your journey to weight loss, Italian style—a commitment to yourself, access to your real feelings, and that connection to your spirit. (Make that four things. I forgot pasta!)

How do you *connect to your spirit?* By honoring that pure and electric being inside of you. In other words, by honoring your true and perfect self. And you *are* perfect. Every goddess is. Perfectly unique. So *celebrate yourself.* And most importantly, *accept yourself.* When you open your eyes in the morning, remind yourself of who and what you are—a part of that creative force behind everything. It's a great way to start the day.

When you plug into your own socket, you don't have to go around trying to plug into someone else's. You create your own juice. And when you're all charged up like that, there's enough in you to light up an auditorium, if not the entire planet. That's *real* energy independence.

Eat Like a Goddess—Divine, Heavenly Meals

You enliven the goddess element in you by nourishing yourself with good food and by doing the things that mean something to you—by living a passionate life that fulfills your dreams. We get into trouble when we try to live up to other people's expectations. A goddess doesn't need anybody else's approval. You're an individual and can't be squeezed into someone else's mold.

How would you act if you knew you were a goddess? For one thing, you'd probably stand up straighter. You'd breathe more deeply, and you'd relax. You could afford to be magnanimous. And you could allow yourself to be ... OUTRAGEOUS!

Most importantly, I'll bet you dollars to doughnuts (or *lira* to *zeppole*) that you'd treat your body like a temple and give it only goddess-level food to eat!

Goddesses Don't Need to Overeat

I believe that, among other things, food issues are intertwined with misplaced passion. When I think back on the hypnotic effect certain foods used to have on me that would throw rationality out the window, I think of how unfulfilled I sometimes felt—all that passion and no place to put it!

Are you a suppressed passionate person? Don't feel bad. Most of us are. And if I spent time with you, I'm sure I could show you some of the places where you're not living fully. It's not your fault. Normally, we're not encouraged to run with our passions. We're told to knuckle down, buckle down, suppress our natural drives and put our noses to someone else's grindstone. So you end up stuffing your passion and stuffing yourself instead.

That's crazy to Italians, who like to find ways to skirt the rules and know that if you give yourself a life filled with passion you'll be less tempted to console yourself with food. It's all about emotional gratification and making life a more enriching experience by tapping into the things that make you feel alive.

In my own case, I broke free of the hypnotic effect that some foods had on me by replacing it with something better. I allowed myself to go to Italy, to sing, dance, and indulge in my real passions. Instead of starving, I found what nourished me, like good food—real food that left my body satisfied. And I learned how to feed my spirit with what nourished my soul—beauty, esthetics, culture, and art.

I made a conscious decision to be true to myself and my inner fun-loving goddess. I stopped being a stiff and allowed myself to play. Can you open up to your own spontaneity a little and stop worrying so much about what everybody else thinks? I'm not talking about becoming an obnoxious attention-seeker who wants the limelight at everyone else's expense. I'm just talking about *being yourself—without apology*. It's enormously freeing, and much more satisfying than a cream puff.

But first you have to *know yourself.* The real you, minus the mask.

Have you become too serious just trying to hold things together? The concept of "holding on" can be a metaphor for hanging onto unnecessary weight, too. Try letting go and just being silly once in a while. It breaks the ice—yours and everyone else's. It lifts the heaviness and gets the party rolling. Tap into your natural playfulness and throw on the liveliness button. We do have a switch that we can turn on and off. The problem is that if you're like most people, yours has been taped into the off position.

Still wondering how to let the goddess out? Well, you're the star of your own life, so allow yourself to be the diva. Can you spice up your wardrobe? Do your current clothes make you feel like a million bucks? A star doesn't wear drab, dowdy clothes that were popular a hundred years ago. How do your clothes make you feel? Are you wearing things better suited to hiding under a rock than being in the spotlight? What if the paparazzi suddenly show up?

One stylish dress and a new pair of shoes (maybe red?) should do it. Paying homage to your inner goddess will actually *save* you money. No more running up the credit cards to make up for emptiness and a lack of passion.

If you've forgotten how to turn on your aliveness, here are my suggestions for throwing the switch.

My Inner Goddess Knows Flamenco!

Goddesses love to dance, because it sends them into bliss. It's good for the heart, the body, and the social life. Plus it melts off pounds.

Before my Italy incarnation, I lived in Japan for a while. I was struggling to keep my sanity in a culture that doesn't exactly encourage you to pull out the stops. (Japan has its charms, but passionate living isn't at the top of the list.) I was dying for lack of a creative outlet. Fortunately, my inner lifeline kicked into action when I happened to see a flamenco version of the opera, *Carmen*. I was captivated by the dancing, the sensuality, and the *passion*. I *had* to take flamenco lessons. It was one of the best decisions I've ever made. This is the positive side of giving in to your passion.

Flamenco allowed me to reach deep inside myself for a beauty and expressiveness I didn't even know I had. It gave me poise, and the live guitar music thrilled me. When I stood before the mirror in my long black skirt, castanets, and red flamenco shoes, I became Carmen— along with twenty inspired and enlivened Japanese Carmens, moving in unison. It was an intoxicating experience and such good exercise!

When I moved to New York, I discovered mambo. I was in divorce hell by this time, and the only thing that got my mind off it was the electrifying Latin music and the thrill of learning to move my body in a new and sensual way. A by-product was that it also provided a nonthreatening way of meeting and interacting with men during a time when I felt fragile. Yes, there were Italian men in the dance class. (You didn't think I'd find them doing the Hokey Pokey, did you?)

There was no mambo, let alone tarantella, when I moved back to California, but there I discovered salsa dancing and later, tango. Both are great for burning calories, and you never have to be alone for long when you're involved in the dance world. Partner dancing, as one of my teachers put it, is "the three-minute romance." It's also been referred to as "the vertical expression of the horizontal desire." But aside from that, one of the best parts is that you get to dress up and be a goddess for the evening.

And if you're afraid to take a dance class, you can always just turn on the music in your living room and dance up a freestyle storm. Which brings us to …

The Spaghetti Dance

Even many Italians don't know about the Spaghetti Dance, but it's happening in pots and pans all across Italy, even as we speak. (I'd like to say I invented it, but I know what happened to Al Gore when he talked about the Internet!)

You know how kung fu moves are inspired by things in nature? So is this dance. It was inspired by the graceful, then increasingly energetic movements of strands of spaghetti as they become agitated and then begin to gyrate spasmodically in a pot of boiling water.

It came to me one day as I was staring into a spaghetti pot. No, actually, I was standing in my living room with a backache from sitting at my computer. I was listening to some music, and I found myself starting to sway and move my body in some of those slow, undulating movements like the kind spaghetti makes as it loosens up and starts to come alive as the water returns to a boil. This dance creates a beautiful, natural, and rhythmic flow that releases stress, energizes all your sleeping parts, and makes you laugh, even if no one else is in the room. It releases your spine and enlivens your entire being.

The Spaghetti Dance is real. Try it. Your body will love it. It's fine to laugh as you're doing it. Just don't laugh at the dance. And as you become accustomed to looking and feeling silly, you'll be ready to attempt your first dance class.

Here's how it's done:

- Turn on some Italian music—preferably the kind that starts out slowly, then picks up speed. Italian music was all the craze in the 1950s, so check out an oldies station on the radio or recordings at your local music store or library.
- Stand limp (like cooked spaghetti), with your knees slightly bent.
- Let your arms and hands hang loose, and then kind of sway from foot to foot to the music, letting your body move gracefully, like a strand of spaghetti just awakening to the undulating movement of the water.
- As you continue to sway, your arms move loosely overhead and down. Be like a rag doll while still swaying.
- Let your pelvis go forward and allow your spine to follow, so that it moves in a serpentine "S" shape.

Do that for a while, and as the music warms up, let your body move in any way that feels good. Let it lead you. Finally, you can pick up speed and just shake it all out in a frenzy. If you need inspiration or find these instructions hard to visualize, it's helpful to observe real spaghetti boiling in a pot.

If you *still do*n't get it, eat the spaghetti, have a sip of wine, and go out and dance under the stars. It hardly gets more goddessy than that!

Learn from Pavarotti

Deep down every one of us is a Renaissance person with many skills and talents. But you have to grant yourself permission to do new things and have the courage to try them. Many of us don't bother because we think in terms of limitations rather than possibilities. Do yourself a favor and come out of your box.

Every time I listen to Pavarotti, I'm moved to tears. And I'm so thankful that he devoted his life to singing. As the son of a baker, he could have just become another baker and deprived the world of his voice. Fortunately for us, he didn't do that. He fought a life-long battle with his weight, by the way. People gossiped about it in opera circles, and it made headlines when he went on a diet. But he didn't let that stop him. He had a mission in life, and he fulfilled it. How many of us can say the same?

You don't have to be Pavarotti to enjoy flexing your vocal muscles. All it takes is deciding that you're going to and then finding a teacher. All my life I wanted to learn how to sing, but I never allowed myself the luxury. Then one day I was sitting in a restaurant in Rome and happened to ask the waiter if he knew how to get to the opera house. Did he know? His eyes bugged out, and he told me he used to sing there every day. Then he burst into song right there in front of me. When he was done, he fixed me with a stare, pointed a finger at my face and said, "You must sing opera."

It had never occurred to me that I could do that. I asked him if it was hard. He shrugged and said, "You have voice, you sing. No have voice, no sing."

When I got back to Manhattan, I was walking down Broadway when I ran into a friend of mine who gushed about recently joining a singing school. I told him what the waiter had said in Rome, and he laughed and said I should take lessons, too. I took his advice. I just went down to the school and signed up. And it was one of the most fun and thrilling things I've ever done.

If you've never learned to sing, you might explore it as another passionate pursuit that taps into your bliss so you're not so dependent on food to give you fake fulfillment. Singing makes you happy! If you can't afford group or private lessons, join a choral group.

Be Your Own Da Vinci

I loved to draw and paint when I was a child. In fact, I wanted to be an artist when I grew up and was even going to do a junior year abroad and study art in Florence. But I ended up going to Washington, D.C. and becoming a journalist instead.

Ever since, from time to time my inner artist has rattled her cage, and I've gotten out my paints and painted just for the pleasure of it. It's absorbing and therapeutic. My painter friend, Anne Deidre Smith, inspired me to pick up my paints again not so long ago, and I couldn't put my brushes down. My attempts were not masterpieces, but they weren't supposed to be. I was just exploring for my own enjoyment.

Try pulling out some watercolors or acrylics and just experimenting with some brush strokes on paper. (Or oils, but they're kind of messy.) Explore and see how satisfying it is. It will open up new avenues of joy and expressiveness. And when you're playing around with the colors, you'll be doing your own version of color therapy.

Really, it's true.

And Why Are We Doing This?

It may sometimes feel that being so focused on weight loss is a rather self-involved, egocentric thing to do. But in case you're not aware of it, there's a bigger picture behind the dream of losing weight. Yes, of course, you should lose weight for yourself. You want to feel good and live a long, healthy life. And looking as if you stepped off the cover of Italian *Vogue* is pretty terrific, too.

But there's an even more important reason. Lose the weight so that you can *become a beacon of hope* for others. "If she can do it, I can do it" is a gift that you give to each person in your life who sees that you are able to achieve a healthy weight by living like an Italian, not dieting like an American.

But wait —there's more still. What are you going to say when it's all over and you have your life review? That you couldn't be bothered reaching your potential because you were too busy having a hot fudge sundae? We all came here for a reason. Lose the weight so you can focus on developing your special talent. The world needs it, and you may be denying it because of your issues with the extra pounds you carry. Don't die without discovering and sharing your unique gift with the world.

Much of life's joy and "juice" is tied up in the pursuit of your passion or talent. Your weight, literally and figuratively, stands between you and your joy. When you can't connect with a loving, positive sense of self, life is unfulfilling, and that may be causing you to turn to food. From now on, let your passion be your new pleasure. Do what satisfies you for the pure joy of it.

If you don't know what your passion is, do some exploration. Any little step you take toward the fulfillment of your dream or your passion will take the focus off of food and a negative body image. Your weight will become less of an issue. When you're fulfilled and happy, you might not even care about *that* anymore.

You Don't Want to Miss a Thing

When you're living a life you love, there's no room for being disconnected or "unconscious." You don't want to miss a moment. When your passion is engaged, you don't have time to obsess about eating. You might even forget to. It doesn't mean you don't like food, or even love it. But you have more important things to think about than whether that jelly doughnut tastes as good as it looks or whether a pint of rocky road would lift your spirits.

And you have more important things to do, like getting passionate about becoming healthy and learning to cook and eat like an Italian!

Chapter 9:

That's *Amore!*

Omnia vincit amor. (Love conquers all.)
—Virgil

Whatever the problem, love is the answer, not food. So, Venus, my little goddess of love, treat yourself well. You deserve it.

We've been on quite a journey together in this book. We've visited the island of Elba, wandered the streets of Rome and Florence, met the people and tasted the food in Tuscany, and gotten to know the hearts, minds, and passionate spirit of the Italian people. I've told you some of my success story with weight loss, Italian style, and I hope I've inspired you to begin to write your story, too.

I assume that by now you've created your collage. You've started making friends with your body, and you've begun seeing yourself as you wish to be. You've banished junk food from your kitchen and have begun eating so well at meals that you're not tempted to snack. You've begun taking advantage of any wonderful open-air markets in your area. (Perhaps you're even using them as flirting opportunities if you're single.) You're eating with the seasons and loving what you eat.

You're spending more quality time at the table and making eating a social occasion when possible, and you've created an inviting atmosphere for your at-home dining. Maybe you're discovering how to make pasta work for you, and you're falling in love with olive oil, to the point where you put it on everything. (Including your skin. Yes, it makes a nourishing body lotion.)

You're working with your mind, and you're moving throughout the day and adding some fun, enlivening type of exercise to your repertoire. And you're working on your dream and connecting with your passion.

If you keep it up, in six months you'll have a different body, if not a different life. You'll be living La Dolce Vita in your own home town, living and loving like an Italian, with passion, joy, and a slim, trim, healthy body that you're proud to maintain.

It's also okay if you haven't done all these things. You don't need to do everything at once and overwhelm yourself. As Marco Polo learned when he set off for China, a journey of a thousand miles begins with a single step.

And Rome wasn't built in a day!

You can take baby steps. And if you fall down, don't beat yourself up. Just give yourself a *bacio* (kiss) for trying, dust yourself off, and get back in the saddle. (Horseback riding is great exercise.)

Just Desserts

So, what's next on the menu? Food, of course! Now that you've digested the "main course"—weight loss, Italian style—I'm serving up dessert. Well, a dessert of sorts, if you catch my drift. On the following pages, you'll find recipes for two of my favorite indulgences, Italian fantasies that are worth saving calories for.

I'm being a little loose with the word "dessert." In this instance, I want to invoke a passionate playtime meal. The chocolate pasta recipe is actually a savory dish. And after that, something *really* sweet. (And a little hot.)

Chocolate Pasta *Appassionata*

This first recipe was surely something inspired by Venus, the love goddess, herself. Use it to celebrate and spice up your life. It's best enjoyed with someone special, but if that person hasn't appeared yet, put them on your "That's For Me!" collage, and in the meantime, fix it for yourself. You're special, too.

Ingredients:

- 1 small basket cherry tomatoes, halved
- 1 cup fresh basil leaves, sliced
- 2 cloves garlic, minced
- ½ cup highest quality extra virgin olive oil
- ½ teaspoon salt
- 1 10-ounce bag chocolate pasta (from specialty stores or Chocoholics Divine Desserts*)
- 4 ounces flavorful goat cheese

Method:

1. Early in the day, combine the cherry tomatoes, the basil, garlic, olive oil, salt and cheese in a large bowl. Cover and let them "steep."
2. When you're ready to eat, heat water for the chocolate pasta.
3. Cook the pasta according to directions (being careful not to overcook it—chocolate pasta can become mushy.)
4. Drain the pasta and add it to the bowl with the tomato mixture.
5. Lightly toss the ingredients.

Chocolate pasta is not a sweet dish. (It's a pasta dish and will serve as your main course for a fun-filled evening.) You'll have to supply the sweetness yourself. I've thought of that, too, because you can follow it with:

Red Hot Dessert

(As we've learned from the Italians, simplicity is often best.)

Ingredients:

- Red Raspberry Chocolate Body Frosting (from Chocoholics Divine Desserts*)
- You and a Loved One

Method:

1. Open the bottle.
2. Use your imagination.

Just don't eat the entire jar yourself, because

Nothing ever tastes as good as being slender feels!

Now *that's* Italian!

Italian-Style Recipes—FREE

And now that you know how to live and eat like an Italian, I want to give you some insider tips on how to cook like one. Launch your new, healthy love affair with food right this minute by going to www. WeightLossItalianStyle.com/bonus to download your free collection of mouthwatering recipes from my companion book, *Weight Loss, Italian Style! Recipes to Drool Over*. Dig in to tasty pastas, appetizers, soups, salads, desserts, and more.

And while you're there, check out my articles, CDs, and programs. You'll find everything you need to lose weight Italian style.

Arrivederci. Have fun!

www.WeightLossItalianStyle.com.

*To purchase chocolate pasta or Red Raspberry Chocolate Body Frosting, visit <u>www.gourmetchocolate.com</u>. (Tell them Jill sent you!)

About the Author

Writer Jill Hendrickson fell in love with Italy and the Italian way of life when she stumbled off a train in Venice as a college student and spent her first night in the broom closet of a fancy Venetian hotel. She returned two decades later to fulfill her dream of studying Italian, and while on the Isle of Elba and later while living with a cooking teacher in Florence, she discovered the secrets used by Italians to maintain their weight while eating some of the most delicious food on the planet.

Jill earned a Master of Fine Arts degree in writing from Columbia University and has written and edited for newspapers, news services, television, and radio. She began travel writing while working for the *Official Airline Guides* and *TravelAge East* and *TravelAge West* magazines. She has worked for the Associated Press, columnist Jack Anderson, States News Service, *The Japan Times*, Kyodo News Service, and NHK Broadcasting. Her stories have appeared around the world in such publications as *The International Herald Tribune* and the *Asian Wall Street Journal.*

Jill holds a certificate in natural healing from the Academy of Natural Healing in New York and is a member of Slow Food, the international nonprofit organization dedicated to helping people reawaking the joy of eating. She has taught writing at colleges and a university in California, worked closely with transformational teacher and bestselling author Barbara De Angelis, and continues to study with a meditation master in India.

Jill spends her time writing, teaching, and leading others through the process of living, eating, and losing weight Italian style!

BUY A SHARE OF THE FUTURE IN YOUR COMMUNITY

These certificates make great holiday, graduation and birthday gifts that can be personalized with the recipient's name. The cost of one S.H.A.R.E. or one square foot is $54.17. The personalized certificate is suitable for framing and will state the number of shares purchased and the amount of each share, as well as the recipient's name. The home that you participate in "building" will last for many years and will continue to grow in value.

Here is a sample SHARE certificate:

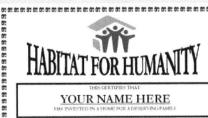

HABITAT FOR HUMANITY

THIS CERTIFIES THAT

YOUR NAME HERE

HAS INVESTED IN A HOME FOR A DESERVING FAMILY

1985-2005

TWENTY YEARS OF BUILDING FUTURES IN OUR
COMMUNITY ONE HOME AT A TIME

1200 SQUARE FOOT HOUSE @ $65,000 = $54.17 PER SQUARE FOOT
This certificate represents a tax deductible donation. It has no cash value.

YES, I WOULD LIKE TO HELP!

I support the work that Habitat for Humanity does and I want to be part of the excitement! As a donor, I will receive periodic updates on your construction activities but, more importantly, I know my gift will help a family in our community realize the dream of homeownership. **I would like to SHARE in your efforts against substandard housing in my community!** *(Please print below)*

PLEASE SEND ME _____ SHARES at $54.17 EACH = $ $_____

In Honor Of: _____

Occasion: (Circle One)   HOLIDAY   BIRTHDAY   ANNIVERSARY

     OTHER: _____

Address of Recipient: _____

Gift From: _____ *Donor Address:* _____

Donor Email: _____

I AM ENCLOSING A CHECK FOR $ $_____ PAYABLE TO HABITAT FOR HUMANITY OR PLEASE CHARGE MY VISA OR MASTERCARD *(CIRCLE ONE)*

Card Number _____ Expiration Date: _____

Name as it appears on Credit Card _____ Charge Amount $ _____

Signature _____

Billing Address _____

Telephone # Day _____ Eve _____

PLEASE NOTE: Your contribution is tax-deductible to the fullest extent allowed by law.
Habitat for Humanity • P.O. Box 1443 • Newport News, VA 23601 • 757-596-5553
www.HelpHabitatforHumanity.org

9 781600 375477